PEDOMETER
WALKING

Other books by Mark Fenton

The Complete Guide to Walking for Health, Weight Loss, and Fitness

Walking Through Pregnancy and Beyond
   (with Lisa Fenton and Tracy Teare)

PEDOMETER
WALKING

Stepping Your Way to Health, Weight Loss, and Fitness

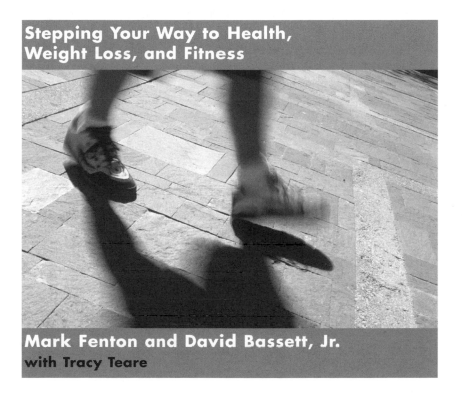

Mark Fenton and David Bassett, Jr.
with Tracy Teare

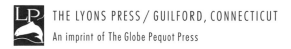

THE LYONS PRESS / GUILFORD, CONNECTICUT

An imprint of The Globe Pequot Press

The Lyons Press is an imprint of The Globe Pequot Press.

10 9 8 7 6

Printed in the United States of America

Book design and composition by Diane Gleba Hall

The following provided photographs for the book: Gary Higgins, pages 6, 36, 86, 87, 94; Mark Fenton, pages 7, 20, 57, 65, 113, 114; David Ellingsen (davidellingsen.com), pages 75, 76, 77; New Lifestyles, page 8; circa 1667 pedometer courtesy of the Museum of the History of Science, University of Oxford, England, page 2.

Library of Congress Cataloging-in-Publication Data

Fenton, Mark.
 Pedometer walking / Mark Fenton and David Bassett, Jr. with Tracy Teare.
   p. cm.
 Includes bibliographical references and index.
 ISBN 978-1-59228-702-4 (alk. paper)
 1. Fitness walking. 2. Weight loss. 3. Physical fitness. I. Bassett, David R.,
   1928- II. Teare, Tracy. III. Title.
RA781.65.F463 2006
613.7'176--dc22

2005028062

To my mom, a dedicated walker,
who often reminds me about the important things in life.

—D.B.

To Joan'd and Fuel, who set me on a joyous adventure
from the very first steps.

—M.F.

". . . the solemn invigorator of the body is exercise, and of all exercises walking is best. A horse gives but a kind of half exercise, and a carriage is no better than a cradle. No one knows, till he tries, how easily a habit of walking is acquired. A person who never walked three miles will in the course of a month become able to walk 15 or 20 without fatigue. . . . Should you be disposed to try it . . . it will be necessary for you to begin with a little, & to increase it by degrees."

—Thomas Jefferson, in a letter
to Thomas Mann Randolf, Jr.
his future son-in-law.
Paris, August 27, 1786

Contents

Acknowledgments

We are indebted to David's colleagues at the University of Tennessee for their contributions to this book. Ed Howley and Dixie Thompson helped shape many of the ideas in the manuscript through discussions and research collaborations. Dr. Diane Klein, a physical activity gerontologist, provided useful information on the effects of aging.

Professors Bruce Craig, Dr. Leroy "Bud" Getchell, and Dr. David Costill had a great impact on David's career, introducing him to human physiology research at Ball State University. At the University of Wisconsin in Madison, Drs. Fran Nagle, Henry Montoye, Jerry Dempsey, and Bill Morgan stimulated his thinking and encouraged him to expand his boundaries. Dr. Barbara Ainsworth, at San Diego State University, offered to serve as a mentor at an early stage of his career.

Drs. Robert Mann, Robert Bligh, and Peter Griffith helped Mark develop his critical thinking and research skills at the Massachusetts

Institute of Technology, and Charles Dillman, Jay Kearney, Leonard Jansen, and too many research assistants to name at the U.S. Olympic Training Center's Sports Science Laboratory were invaluable mentors over the years.

Dr. Catrine Tudor-Locke, at Arizona State University, is a leader in the field of pedometer research and has provided much insight into the field. Dr. Gertrude Huntington introduced David to the Amish, and provided invaluable assistance with that study. David Luthy, of the Heritage Historical Library, kindly offered generous assistance. Dr. Yoshiro Hatano of Kyushu University in Japan, one of the pioneers in this field, has extended friendship, good advice, and words of encouragement.

Thank you to the many graduate students who carried out most of the research and data collection. Their enthusiasm and optimism keeps the research fresh, and it has been a pleasure to observe their accomplishments. We are grateful to Pamela Andrews, a capable laboratory assistant who helped to gather research articles in the library.

Many thanks to Ann Treistman, our acquiring editor at Lyons Press, who saw the value of this book and started our collaboration on the topic. And special appreciation to editor Holly Rubino, whose acumen and tremendous calm allowed her to negotiate the treacherous waters of dealing with a professional journalist, a research scientist, and a strong-willed health advocate. Thanks for her steady hand in seeing this book through.

Lastly, thanks to our families for their patience and support not just in the writing of this book, but in our always time consuming efforts in the research, teaching, and promotion of physical activity. Without them, this book would not be a reality, but thanks to them it has been a joy.

A Safety Reminder

This program promotes physical activity and will encourage you to increase your daily step totals over time. Although the approach is gradual and based on your initial activity level, as with any exercise program there are inherent risks. These risks, such as musculoskeletal injury or cardiorespiratory discomfort or distress, are very low for activities such as moderate-intensity walking. However, the risks tend to be greater for higher-intensity activities and for people who are pregnant, older, or overweight, or who have been inactive or have preexisting conditions. So it's best to check with your doctor before starting this program, even if it's just a phone call to make sure you don't have any reason to restrict your activity levels. That said, your physician is likely to encourage you to simply get walking.

Introduction

Ericka's Incredible Shrinking World

Ericka Kostka is the kind of person some women might envy. She's an attractive blonde with sparkling blue eyes, an easy smile, and quick wit. Plus, she has the kind of trim physique that elicits the jealous response, "Oh, I bet she's never had to diet a day in her life." Of course we all loved Ericka, an editor at *Walking Magazine*. She had that physique in part because she did eat healthfully—although we recall a certain fondness for ice cream during office birthday celebrations. And *diet*, as in the verb? It wasn't in her vocabulary. Turns out she had a much simpler weight control plan—walk 5 to 6 miles a day. And here's the funny thing: It wasn't really a plan.

Ericka didn't own a car and was living in Boston, a 20-minute walk from the subway line that she took to work every day, and 40 minutes from her boyfriend Karl's apartment. So a typical day included at least 40 minutes (easily 4,000 to 5,000 steps) of active commuting for work, frequent neighborhood jaunts on foot for shopping and errands, and regular walks to Karl's.

Then something happened—she and Karl got married, and found a great apartment nearer to the subway. This shrank Ericka's world—she could spend less time commuting, and lots more time with Karl in marital bliss. But it also had the unintended consequence of causing Ericka to start putting on weight. Nothing earth shattering, but she couldn't figure it out—she and Karl were, if anything, eating better because they went out less, and she still went to the gym three or more days a week to lift weights. So why the newly acquired pounds? Wearing a pedometer gave her the answer.

While working at the magazine she had used a pedometer, and she knew her old lifestyle had often required 12,000 steps or more in a day. Wearing it postmarriage informed her that she'd lost a few thousand steps from her daily commute, and often another 5,000 in errands or walking to Karl's. This meant she *wasn't* burning several hundred calories she'd normally expended every day. For a day or two it was no big deal, but five days a week, one week after another, and it added up. In two months, she'd put on five pounds, and feared the trend would continue.

Thankfully, her pedometer gave her the answer—she began hopping off the subway a couple of stops early to inject several thousand steps back into her trip to and from work, and consciously reinserted step-heavy walks for errands during the day. The result: Her weight returned to normal, and she didn't feel she'd had to add a bunch of time-intensive "structured exercises" to her day. Her experience highlights two important lessons.

First, everyone can benefit from using a pedometer, even a professional like Ericka who researches and promotes health and fitness. Pedometer use shines an accurate and unemotional light on your daily activity, and provides a frank assessment of how active you really are.

Second, it's all about your lifestyle. Sure, formal exercise, such as going to a gym or taking a class, is great. But what you do in normal daily life matters tremendously—and can be a great help or a huge hindrance to meeting your health, weight loss, and fitness goals.

This book is built on these two lessons. With America in the throes of an obesity epidemic, with diabetes and chronic disease on a steady rise, we need more than an occasional trip to the gym. We need to look at our daily lives and figure how active we really are—or, in most cases, are not. And then we need solutions—perhaps not the same as Ericka's, but as simple and effective—that get our bodies back in motion and our calories back in balance.

After all, we are a species that is designed to move. From roaming the savanna in search of food as hunter-gatherers to settling down as subsistence farmers struggling to scratch out a harvest, our ancestors lived in a world that demanded lots of physical work just to find their next meal. Even after the industrial revolution, it was common for people to do hard physical labor for as much as 60 hours a week and to use walking as the primary mode of transportation. To put it simply, we've always had to expend calories to get calories.

But that has changed dramatically for most Americans, especially in the last 50 years. Most of us drive for the vast majority of our daily travel, an increasing number of people work in office or service settings, and even manufacturing jobs require less and less actual physical labor and energy expenditure. And a meal of 1,600

Calories—easily three-quarters or more of our daily requirement—can be ordered through the window of a car and consumed in the driver's seat without taking a single step. That's a far cry from having to hunt it down or grow it, as we had to just one or two centuries ago. And that's a huge change in a mere blink of evolutionary time; far too fast for our genes to have kept up and made us more effective calorie burners. The result: a chronic caloric imbalance, with lots of Americans consistently eating more than they expend, and a host of health problems related to sedentary living and obesity. In fact, it's not so much an obesity epidemic as an epidemic of physical inactivity and poor nutrition. Obesity is just the first warning sign, with other chronic conditions following quickly behind.

STEPPING STONE

"A journey of a thousand miles begins with a single step."
LAO-TZU

So we have a few choices. Should we stay on constant and severe diets? Not only is this not too appealing, but based on the sales of diet books, flourishing weight loss programs, and skyrocketing rates of obesity, it's not too successful, either. (Although eating a better diet clearly *is* a priority for most Americans, we won't try to tackle that daunting task in this book.)

How about we go back to our hunter-gatherer roots and chase down our food with spears? Or depend only on what we can grow with our own hands in backyard gardens for our sustenance? Also not likely.

Or perhaps we should find ways to build physical activity back into our daily lives?

This book assumes that you, like Ericka, think this last option would be a good start. By the time you're done reading and have started using a pedometer for at least six weeks, you'll know it's a fantastic idea. After all, our goal is to give you all the information you need to get started on a year-round program designed to improve your health and energy levels, lose weight, and increase your fitness. It's packaged as a six-week plan that's easy to follow and impossible to screw up. But it's really a guide to permanent lifestyle change, not just six weeks of good behavior. It's guaranteed to guide you to adding more activity to your day in the best and most sustainable way.

So a fine way to use the book is to read one section per week as you actually follow the six-week program step by step. If you're really itchy to get that pedometer on your hip, then at least read the 11 most commonly asked questions about pedometer walking (see page 125), which acts as a sort of quick-start guide. But reading and stepping through the full six-week program is what will provide you the best sense of how you're going to make it happen in your life. It may mean going to the gym occasionally or adding other "structured" exercise to your days now and then; or you may do it entirely by tucking incidental activity into your routines. (No doubt eating a healthier diet would also help, and it's a goal well worth your attention.) But it's clear that with bodies this well designed for daily movement, the first and easiest step is to simply *take* more steps.

Week One

How Active Is Your Life?

You read about it in the papers and hear about it on the news. Federal health agencies say it could bust the Medicare trust fund well before Social Security gets into trouble. Your doctor may have even had a few words to say about your personal contribution to it. We're talking about the nation's obesity epidemic, of course.

There's a constant drumbeat telling us that Americans are over-weight and getting heavier. Inevitably, fast food, lousy vending machine offerings, and ballooning portion sizes are part of the dis-cussion. But that's only half of the story. An important half, no doubt—just check out the movie *Super Size Me* or the books *Fast Food Nation* or *Fat Land* for an enthralling and sobering look at the American diet—but there's another side to this equation.

Physical activity—specifically, the lack thereof. Over the past 50 years, technology has made everyday living and working easier, but it's also sapped nearly every chance we have to be physically active. Only a few decades ago, most Americans did not have automatic garage door openers, automatic dishwashers, or computers and e-mail, not to mention cars. Now most do. In a typical day, vast numbers of Americans now walk a few steps to a car, pull up to a drive-through window at a fast-food chain for breakfast, drive to work, take an elevator up to the office, sit at a workstation for eight hours, and then reverse the process—perhaps even including a drive-through dinner and pickup at a video store—to go home. Soon after, we park ourselves in front of the television for the evening, maybe following a spin on the riding lawn mower or an effortless trip to the automatic washer and dryer. All told, that's a lot of sitting. This marked drop in activity affects our daily routines 24/7, and it adds up. As you do less—and eat more, or even just the same amount—those extra calories have nowhere to go, so they get stored as fat.

STEPPING STONE

Leonardo da Vinci once sketched a simple design for a mechanical pedometer. Later European pedometers used a string tied from the belt to the lower leg to record steps. In 1789, Swiss-born watchmaker Abraham-Louis Breguet perfected a self-contained mechanism for use in pedometers.

This pedometer is circa 1667.

Is this relationship between physical inactivity and excessive fat proven? You bet. The evidence mounts, and much of it is tied to the number of steps we take each day. Some of the most compelling work comes from Japanese researcher Dr. Yoshiro Hatano, who began studying pedometer use in the 1960s. He noted that Japanese adults who walked 10,000 steps per

STEPPING STONE

How Do Pedometers Work?

If you're one of those curious types who just has to know how gadgets do their magic, read on. Otherwise, consider yourself warned: *techy-details ahead.*

A pedometer is a pager-sized device with a clip that attaches to your belt or waistband. It's worn on your hip, senses your body's movement, and measures how many steps you take. Pedometers basically use three different types of mechanisms to record steps. Most new electronic pedometers have a horizontal, spring-suspended lever arm that bounces up and down with each step. This movement opens and closes an electrical circuit, which causes the number of steps to be counted. These pedometers are more reliable than the old mechanical step counters, which used a ratchet-and-gear mechanism for counting steps.

A second type of pedometer uses a magnetic reed proximity switch. This pedometer has a horizontal lever arm, with a tiny magnet on the end. When the magnet moves past a glass-enclosed reed switch, it attracts a flexible piece of metal inside. This closes the switch and records one step. A third type of pedometer uses a device that measures acceleration, and it's a good choice if you do a combination of walking and running. This accelerometer determines how much energy you put into a given activity. It has a flexible beam that resembles a diving board with a weight on the end. As you walk, the beam flexes slightly up and down, compressing a piezoelectric crystal and producing an electric current. The currents are used to count steps and predict calorie expenditure.

day had less stored fat, compared with those who walked less. Similar relationships have been shown in the United States. One study found that women who took at least 10,000 steps per day were in the normal weight range, and weighed considerably less than women who averaged 6,000 to 10,000 steps a day; women accumulating fewer than 6,000 steps a day were heavier still.

STEPS TO SUCCESS
Don't Count on a Cheap Pedometer's Count

McDonald's introduced a "Stepometer" with a salad and bottled water in a promotional Go Active Happy Meal in May 2004. It may be no coincidence that this promotion, which ran through July 2004, launched within days of the introduction of the movie *Super Size Me*, an entertaining but biting indictment of the fast-food industry's menus and marketing practices (see page 25). The positive result, however, is that between 10 and 15 million pedometers were snapped up, and many stores ran out of them before the end of the promotion.

Dr. Weimo Zhu, a professor at the University of Illinois at Urbana-Champaign, was the senior scientist on a study that tested the accuracy of McDonald's pedometers. They had subjects repeatedly walk exactly 100 steps with the pedometers, and found that the worst ones displayed mean steps ranging from 42 to 129; the best one ranged from 98 to 120. The study concluded, "Due to inaccuracy and inconsistency in step counting and poor instrument equivalence, McDonald's Stepometers have no merit in promoting physical activities."

Similar results have been recorded with the promotional pedometers included inside specially marked boxes of Kellogg's cereal. Yet the outcome of these promotions wasn't all negative. Michael Wortley, a sales clerk at the Runner's Market in Knoxville, Tennessee, reported that the week after the McDonald's promotion started, people started coming into the store asking for a better pedometer to replace their Go Active Stepometer. Internet vendors of pedometers also reported an increase in sales, likely due to all the publicity.

Some experts viewed the food industries' interest in promoting physical activity as an attempt to deflect charges that they are part of the problem behind the obesity crisis. At least the general public seemed to recognize the benefits of measuring steps; unfortunately, they were frustrated by the inaccuracies of the cheap promotional devices. It serves as a reminder that it's worth investing in a good-quality, accurate pedometer, and even trying it out in the store before buying if you have any doubts at all about performance.

Other studies continue to confirm that inactivity is connected to ill health. Recent research led by Dr. Lawrence Frank at the University of Vancouver, British Columbia, found that the risk of obesity rises 6 percent with each additional hour per day spent in a car. Another study in 2003 concluded that watching two or more hours of television a day increases your risk of diabetes by more than 10 percent and of obesity by nearly 25 percent. So clearly one of the best ways to reduce your chances of severe obesity and re-lated chronic diseases is to be physically active and reduce your sedentary time. And as you'll soon see, the pedometer is just the tool to help you be aware of how much you're sitting versus stepping.

Where to Get a Pedometer

Most sporting goods or specialty athletic retailers (such as running or outdoor gear stores) carry pedometers, but they are also available online from a number of Internet companies. See the Resources section at the end of the book for online vendors.

Pedometers typically range in price from $15 to $30, with fancier models with lots of memory (able to store days' worth of steps) costing more, and some simple mechanical (or analog) models being even cheaper. A mechanical step counter will likely be less accurate at reliably counting your steps and more likely to be confused by nonstep movements (say, a bouncy ride in a car).

Since accuracy is really important when you're counting steps, consider getting a simple digital model. Some pedometers estimate the distance you walk and the calories you burn, but they generally cost more and you don't really need those features. A simple digital step counter with a numerical LCD (liquid crystal diode, as on most digital watches) readout and a single button to reset the step count to zero at the end of the day is all you need. A Japanese company called Yamax makes Digi-Walkers—sold in the United States under several brand names—and these were among the most accurate in research tests; they have a steps-only version for about $25 retail.

Also look for a really solid clip for your belt—not a flimsy one that will snap off easily and allow your pedometer to end up in the toilet. (Trust us, it happens all the time.) Even better, get one with a small safety cord that you can pass through a belt loop or clip to your waistband. Manufacturers regularly improve their models or introduce new ones, so we can't recommend a definitive best pick. But there is a listing of many currently available models in the Resources section at the end of this book.

STEPS TO SUCCESS

Reading a Clock-Face Pedometer

A less expensive but easy-to-use style of analog (mechanical) pedometer—often sold in bulk for $5 to $10 each, and used in workplace or health care activity promotion programs—has a clock face with a long and a short hand, and numerals from 1 to 10 on the dial. You point both hands up to the 10 to start, for a reading of zero. As the long hand goes around clockwise, it counts hundreds of steps (like minutes), while the short hand moves at one-tenth the speed and counts thousands of steps (like hours). If your goal is 10,000 steps a day, then the task is straightforward—simply get the short hand to circle the dial once, and you've collected 10,000.

At lesser totals, it's easy to read where you are. First look at the short hand, and figure out what thousand you're on, then get the hundreds and tens from the long hand.

Can you read the step total on this clock-face pedometer? If you said 8,280, then you're on the mark.

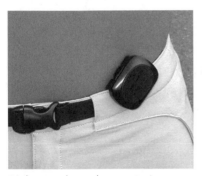

To wear the pedometer correctly, align it with one knee.

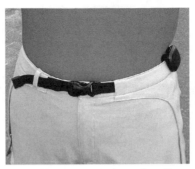

This pedometer is much too far off to the side.

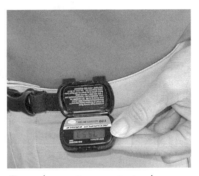

Make sure the pedometer isn't twisted like this.

To read your step count, simply open the pedometer case.

How to Wear a Pedometer

Wear a pedometer on the front of your waist, in line with one knee. Not in the middle under your belly button, and not off to side where cowboys have their holsters. Have it on the front of your body, but just off to one side; which side is up to you.

Make sure the pedometer is held straight up and down and is flat against your body—it shouldn't be twisted to the left or right, nor should it be leaning forward or back. This can be a problem for folks who are high waisted or wear their pants pulled way up,

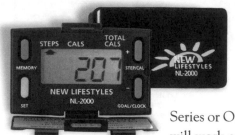

or whose belly bulges enough to lean the pedometer forward. (A possible solution: If you're more than 40 pounds overweight, you could use the New Lifestyles NL Series or Omron HJ-112 pedometers, which will work even when tilted.)

Reset the pedometer to zero, and simply walk around a little bit while actually counting the steps taken by both feet. After you've counted 50 or more steps, check the pedometer and see if it agrees with your count. If you and the pedometer are within five steps, you're in good shape. (It's okay if it's not exactly the same as your count. The pedometer may have registered an extra step when you closed it, or missed a tiny shuffle step that you counted.) However, if you find an error that's greater than 10 percent, test it again. If the error is recurring, return the pedometer and get another.

Steps Matter

Even a modest number of steps spread over the day or week can make a difference. To illustrate this, imagine your weight has been stable, but because of a change in jobs you had to eliminate your 20-minute round-trip walk to the bus stop, five days a week. You'd lose about a half mile or 1,000 steps every morning and evening, Monday through Friday. Over a year, if you didn't change anything else—didn't change what you eat, didn't increase or decrease your exercise level otherwise—you'd gain two to three pounds. A few pounds in one year; doesn't sound like much, right? But do that for 10 to 15 years in a row, and you're 30 pounds overweight—enough for a person of average height to be considered medically obese.

What's more, Americans typically gain about two pounds each year of adulthood—a rate that clearly can be explained by a very small but consistent decrease in daily steps over time.

The point is that you need to be aware of these seemingly benign shifts in activity—they do add up, and they do affect your waistline. And not just your waistline—people who are insufficiently active are at an elevated risk for a disturbingly long list of afflictions from diabetes and cardiovascular disease to osteo-porosis, clinical depression, and a growing list of cancers. Amaz-ingly enough, losing steps every day could lead to losing several years of life span.

That's the bad news. The good news is simple: A pedometer can help you monitor even small changes in activity level, can alert

 PEDOMETER PRO

Thomas Jefferson: A Walker Ahead of His Time

When he wasn't busy establishing our new democracy or penning the Declaration of Independence, Thomas Jefferson was out walking. "The solemn invigorator of the body is exercise, and of all exercises walking is best," he wrote to his future son-in-law in 1786. He would be adored by health experts the world over for his words: "Not less than two hours a day should be devoted to exercise, and the weather should be little regarded. . . ."

Jefferson was also sold on pedometers, and is often unduly credited with inventing the device. In fact, he bought his in France, where he walked to landmarks all over Paris, carefully recording the number of steps in his notebook. An all-season walker, he noted that covering a mile in summer required 2,066.5 steps, while the "brisk walk of winter" reduced it to 1,735 steps. Clearly he didn't let the cold weather stop him; Jefferson simply picked up the pace (and extended his stride—a natural result of faster walking) to keep warm. Not a bad suggestion for the rest of us, in fact.

Lee Gets a Little Too Excited, Too Soon

While filming the PBS series *America's Walking*, we gave a number of people pedometers to chart their experiences. Their instructions were clear, and identical to this program: Wear the pedometer all day every day and record your steps. For the first week, don't change your life at all, and *don't try for any additional exercise.* Then after getting a baseline measurement of your activity levels, set some goals and begin working to boost your daily steps. Eventually, try to meet or exceed the goal of 10,000 steps a day.

One of the volunteers, Lee Vickers from Scituate, Massachusetts, was really jazzed to be in the program, and looked forward to figuring out how to get more activity into her days. She'd launched a new business the previous year, had found getting out for regular exercise a struggle, and had seen her weight start to climb. But like many people, she'd heard the recommendation that walking at least 10,000 steps per day would improve her long-term health prospects and help with weight control. In fact, she was so excited to have her new pedometer that we saw her out for a walk at 6:00 AM on Wednesday, the third day of the program.

Now, although we understood her enthusiasm, that was *exactly* the wrong thing to do. Here's why: It could give her a false sense of her typical activity levels, and then cause her to set her future step goals unreasonably high. It's important that your first week really be as representative as possible of your normal life. If you usually laze around and watch sports on weekends, then do that this week; if you usually spend hours gardening, then garden away. If you normally get up and walk at 6:00 AM, then keep doing it; but if you normally sleep until 7:30, stick with that routine.

For Lee, it was important that she learn how busy, but not necessarily active, her new business had made her. So don't make the same mistake—for the first week, forget you've got the pedometer on at all, and learn how active you really are.

you when you need to accommodate for them, and can be a wonderfully effective motivational tool. But first you have to measure your current baseline of activity.

Patience, Grasshopper. First, Find Your Baseline.

To use your pedometer most effectively, we recommend a bit of forbearance and patience—exactly one week's worth. When you know how active you are initially, your pedometer becomes a valuable motivator as you track your progress and gradually increase the number of steps you take each day. So before we sell you on the benefits of adding more steps to your days, here's a look at how you'll use the pedometer for the first week. Detailed instructions and a recording log are found at the end of this section. Each subsequent section of the book covers another week of pedometer use.

The goal the first week is to get a baseline measurement of your physical activity level. To put it simply, wear your pedometer all day every day for a full week. (Why a full week instead of just a few days? Because activity levels can vary a lot from day to day depending on work and play, weekdays versus weekends, and even the weather.)

This is important: During this baseline measurement, try not to change your normal routine at all; neither increase nor decrease your typical daily activity. This is not the week to sign up with a personal trainer or to join a health club. In fact, don't think about the pedometer at all—just put it on first thing in the morning and take it off at night. Wear it for everything you do except when you're immersed in water or naked. (We won't get into the challenges of pedometer use while naked.) Only look at the step count once a day—when you take the pedometer off at bedtime and record your step total for the day. Then reset the pedometer to zero

STEPPING STONE

How Many Steps Do Americans Get?

We don't know for sure how many steps per day the average American takes, though it's of increasing interest to researchers and government health agencies. In the meantime, the following numbers from a study of 1,000 adults in Colorado give us a snapshot:

- 33 percent take less than 5,000 steps per day.
- 29 percent take 5,001 to 7,500 steps per day.
- 22 percent take 7,501 to 10,000 steps per day.
- 16 percent take more than 10,000 steps per day.

So more than half of Coloradans averaged between 5,000 and 10,000 steps a day. And because data from the Centers for Disease Control show that Colorado residents are among the most active in the nation, it's a safe bet that many of us lag behind these levels.

for the next day and go to sleep. You get the picture: Wear it daily, and for now don't think about how many steps you're taking.

The Sometimes Shocking Difference Between *Busy* and *Active*

Our days are so jam-packed that to describe them as busy is an understatement. But even though you may feel like you've run a marathon by bedtime, chances are you're actually doing very little in the way of true physical activity. Think about it. If you work at a desk job—even part time—and spend the rest of your day preparing meals, ferrying children, and overseeing laundry, baths, and bedtimes, or dashing to meetings and social and civic obligations, you're still sitting for the majority of the day. Frustratingly few of the things that consume time in modern life have anything to do with being physically active. Our exhaustion has more to do with the frantic pace of our lives than with actual exercise.

The challenge, then, is to find ways to add physical activity to your routine without further taxing your busy schedule. It can be done. First, know that you can count lots of things that you might not currently recognize as exercise. As a general rule, activities that require substantial and frequent movements of your major muscle groups—legs, torso, arms, shoulders—count. To illustrate this, here's a quick look at activities that do and don't qualify:

The Difference Between Busy and Active

Keeps You *Busy*	Keeps You *Active*
Driving to four shopping centers to do four errands.	Walking to four downtown stores to do four different errands.
Changing a diaper, reading, to, feeding a child.	Playing tag, going for a walk, doing the Hokey Pokey with a child.
Answering 16 e-mails.	Taking the stairs up six flights to talk with a real person.
Sitting in stalled traffic.	Riding your bike instead of driving.
Paying bills.	Picking up, dusting, and vacuuming the living room. Fast.
Driving kids to softball, the dentist, and band practice.	Running drills and chasing down balls at softball practice.
Preparing meals; washing dishes.	Weeding the garden; washing the car.

Not surprisingly, those things that contribute to real activity (the right-hand column in the table) will build your daily step total; those things that just keep you busy may wear you down and tire you out, but they don't add many steps to your day. That's the

Joe Learns How Active He Really Is (Not)

Joe is a friend of ours who drove a limousine in the Boston area. He'd enjoyed sports and been active as a child and young man, but found that driving had added a few pounds to his formerly fit frame. Despite that, he laughed when he learned that research had shown many people, especially office workers and those living in car-oriented suburbs, get fewer than 5,000 or even 3,000 steps in a day. In not so many words, he asked how anyone still living could be that sedentary. And he was certain that he got at least 5,000 steps a day, if only from romping with his kids each evening.

So we gave him a pedometer and challenged him not to change his life at all, but just to measure his steps on some typical workdays.

To say he was surprised does not do justice to the word. On one particularly notable day with lots of driving jobs, he found he'd gotten only 1,800 steps, which is less than a mile of walking! Joe was absolutely flabbergasted—how could he be so busy, end the day so utterly wiped out, and yet have gotten so little physical activity? And no doubt his work—the stress of driving in Boston traffic, urgent calls, and sometimes frantic clients—is exhausting. But hours in the car seat meant very little time for any real movement at all.

Joe's solution? Well, he's moved on to other work now, but he found that an intermediate step was to simply get out of the car and walk absolutely anytime he was waiting on a fare or call. His cell phone kept him in touch with the dispatcher, and he even began building a list of favorite places to wait for calls, such as the East Boston waterfront path near Logan Airport. In the end, he decided the job was too sedentary for his health—and we'd like to think that the pedometer helped spur him on to more active pursuits.

beauty of a pedometer: It tells you when a busy day is only masquerading as an active one.

The next step is to find ways to make time for activity, and there are as many ways to tackle this as there are people in the world.

They range from the mundane—such as using the bathroom on the next floor up at work or school—to the life altering, like moving to a community where the physical environment encourages walking to schools, shops, and work. But first, you've got to make a bit of a mental shift and recognize physical activity as something of value, all on its own, and not simply a means to fitting into your favorite jeans.

Physical Activity Is Its Own Reward

When you think *exercise*, are you really just thinking *weight control*? You're not alone. And though obesity is no small problem in America, the benefits of physical activity go well beyond weight loss. In addition to looking better and preventing creeping pounds, you can expect these rewards with regular, moderate exercise:

- More energy.
- Less stress, depression, and anxiety.
- Less body fat.
- Increased HDL cholesterol (the good kind).
- Reduced blood pressure.
- Sounder sleep.
- Better immune function.
- Healthier blood glucose levels.
- Reduced risk for chronic diseases, from osteoporosis to cancer.

If that's not enough, there's no shortage of evidence that modest amounts of walking can increase longevity. Walking has been linked to a reduction in coronary heart disease (CHD) deaths in both men and women. Through the 1990s, the Honolulu Heart

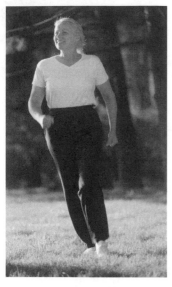

Program examined 2,900 retired men of Japanese ancestry over a period of seven years. In that study, men who reported walking at least 1.5 miles per day were only half as likely to die from heart attacks, compared with their less active peers. Cancer rates were also lower among the more active men.

Similarly impressive results have been seen in large-scale studies of women. In 1999, the renowned Nurses' Health Study found that women who walked more than three hours per week at a brisk pace had a 35 percent decrease in heart attack risk. More recently, Dr. I-Min Lee and her colleagues at Harvard University found that even getting out the door to walk for at least one hour per week—an average of just under 10 minutes a day—

 STEPPING STONE

A New Tool to Rein in High Blood Pressure

A study at the University of Tennessee found that a pedometer-based walking program can help you control your blood pressure. Dr. Dixie Thompson and her graduate students had sedentary women with moderately high blood pressure increase the amount of walking they did; on average they increased from 5,400 steps to 9,700 steps per day. Over six months, the group showed a drop of 11 points in their resting, systolic blood pressure readings. Though no instructions about dieting were given, the women also lost an average of three pounds. None of these changes were seen in the control group, who were not instructed to increase their steps.

STEPS TO SUCCESS

The Perfect Job for Stepping

Researcher Maria Sequeira studied Swiss citizens to get a snapshot of average step counts for a variety of careers and occupations in an eight-hour day. Don't be surprised if your totals are substantially higher or lower than typical for your profession. From looking at a variety of data, it's clear that there can be an incredible amount of variation. For example, in one study, some housewives took 3,000 steps in 24 hours, while others took 11,000. It's not hard to see that this can occur in a number of occupations. One nurse, for example, might sit at a desk running a call center, and another might be zipping from room to room, on her feet all day. The point is that the data provides a general sense of the wide range of activity among different occupations, and illustrates how little activity sedentary jobs afford. It also indicates that it's well worth using a pedometer to get a sense of how active you are during a typical eight-hour workday.

- Manufacturing and assembly worker, 960 average steps.
- Telephone operator, 2,400 average steps.
- Hairdresser, 3,280 average steps
- Painter, 7,120 average steps.
- Laborer, 10,560 average steps.
- Postal carrier, 13,280 average steps.
- Restaurant server, 16,160 average steps.

Looks like if you can stand the heat, waiting tables would be a sure way to logging lots of daily steps and getting healthy. (Unless the chef's desserts became a temptation . . .)

women saw a modest decrease in the risk of heart disease. The benefits were the same regardless of pace.

Enough studies have connected being physically active with a reduced risk for cancer that the American Cancer Society lists a sedentary lifestyle as a risk factor for cancer right alongside smoking. In fact, an expert panel of the International Agency for Research on Cancer (of the World Health Organization) estimates a 20 to 40 percent reduction in the risk of breast cancer for the most physically active women. A recent report on women who had already been *diagnosed* with the disease even measured as much as a 50 percent reduction in the risk of death for those who walked three to five hours a week at a moderate pace, compared with less active women. So adding more steps may be helpful in both preventing and fighting disease.

Despite the impressive stack of proof that shows walking can help you live a healthier, longer life, it will probably be the less tangible thing that hooks you once you start: quality of life. The first

STEPPING STONE
Age Matters

American researcher Catrine Tudor-Locke reports in her delightful booklet *Manpo-Kei: The Art and Science of Step Counting* that typical daily step totals tend to differ depending on your age. Again, these are just average ranges, and you may well fall outside them.

- 8- to 10-year-old children: 12,000 to 16,000 steps per day.
- Healthy, younger adults (age 20 to 40): 7,000 to 13,000 steps per day.
- Healthy older adults (age 50 to 70): 6,000 to 8,500 steps per day.
- Adults living with chronic illness or disability: 3,500 to 5,500 steps per day.

That said, our experience is that we are seeing increasing numbers of Americans with totals at the low end or well below these "typical" ranges, so it's likely the group averages are drifting downward even as you read!

thing walkers often mention—even if they've walked off more than 100 pounds, or walked away from serious health threats—is how good they feel about themselves. Walkers frequently report the good vibes of reduced stress, improved mood, growing self-confidence, and a sense of empowerment. They talk about how their walking time is essential to keeping a sense of balance in their lives. Some use this time to plan, unwind, socialize with a friend, or just plain get away from it all. And whether they become avid hikers or racers or stick with a regimen of 10,000 steps a day, the key is that they believe in themselves as physical, capable people. You may start clipping on that pedometer to burn more calories, but you'll probably want to keep it on for the feel-good factor that comes with being active.

Week One Program

The routine for this program is simple, and all the instruction you need you get on the very first day. Here it is:

- Wear the pedometer daily, from rising in the morning until bed at night, except when you're immersed in water.
- Wear it on the front of your waist and align it with your left or right knee. Do not wear it in the middle under your belly button, nor off to the side near your hipbone, but rather on the front of your body, just off to one side.
- Make sure the pedometer faces up and down—it shouldn't be twisted to the left or right, nor should it be leaning forward or back. This might present a problem for anyone who is high waisted or wears his or her pants pulled way up, or whose belly tips the pedometer forward.
- Put the pedometer on first thing in the morning, wear it all

STEPPING STONE

In Japan, running postmen called *Hikyaku* or "flying legs" wore pedometers in the 17th through 19th centuries. Like our Pony Express, they handed off mail to other runners, each covering as many as 60 to 90 miles in a day with bundles of letters carried on sticks over their shoulders.

day, and take it off at night as you climb into bed. When you take it off, read the total number of steps for the day, write them down (you can use the step log provided here), and then reset the pedometer to zero so you're ready for tomorrow.

- As you write down your step total for the day, also make a brief note of anything unusual that might have especially affected your step total. Nothing elaborate—just note any real step boosters ("car broke down, walked to work" or "kid's field trip") or step stealers ("sick, stayed home").

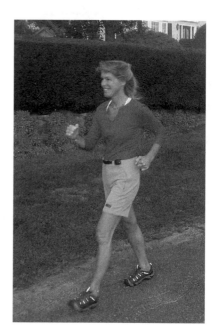

- At the end of seven days, add up your daily counts, divide by 7, and you have your average daily steps for the week.

A reminder: If you're not sure the pedometer is reading properly, do this simple test. Reset the pedometer to zero, and simply walk around a little bit while actually counting the steps of both feet in your head. After you've counted 50 or more steps, check the pedometer and see if it agrees with your count. If you and the pedometer are within five steps, you're in good shape. (It's okay if it's not exactly the same as your count. The pedometer may have registered an extra step when you closed it, or missed a tiny shuffle step that you counted.)

Finally, you have special instructions for just this first week of the program, based on the fact that you want to learn your baseline activity level, a measure of how many steps you take in normal daily life. Don't look at the pedometer readout during the day. Don't open it, don't even think about it. If there's no hinged cover, then cover the readout with black tape. Simply forget you've got your pedometer on, until you take it off at the end of the day to record the total. Certainly exercise if you typically do, but don't *add* any exercise to your routine this week—that can give a false sense of your regular activity levels.

Week One Step Log

Number of steps	Anything special today?
Monday	
Tuesday	
Wednesday	
Thursday	
Friday	
Saturday	
Sunday	
Week Total	

Daily average: _____
(total steps for the week divided by 7)

Daily goal for next week: _____
(daily average x 1.2, for a 20% increase)

Week Two

Finding Steps in Everyday Life

L ike you couldn't see this coming: Our first bit of advice is the key
to why pedometers are so fantastic. Your goal this week is
to start small—really small. So small that you're absolutely sure to
succeed. Your goal is to increase your average daily steps over the
first week by only 20 percent. Don't shoot for the moon, don't
prove what a great athlete you are (or once were). Just find enough
minutes of walking every day to average 20 percent more steps a
day this week than you did last week. And have faith that we're
leading you down a road that's going to get you where you want to
go—great health, weight loss, lots more energy, and a new modeling career with lots of magazine covers.

Okay, maybe not the modeling career. But for now, stick with the 20 percent increase in your steps, and we promise the other three will come.

Add Steps Almost Effortlessly

With a few subtle shifts in routine, it's easy to convert inactivity to activity, and significantly boost the total number of steps you take each day. You can easily cover 100 steps in one minute of continuous activity. Make it a purposeful walk—trying to get somewhere fast—and you'll add 120 to 130 steps per minute or more. Those minutes add up, and the opportunity to use them comes up all the time. The trick is to take advantage of them throughout the day.

Dr. Andrea Dunn, a former researcher at the Cooper Institute for Aerobics Research and a pedometer fan, had an interesting take on this. One recommendation she used to give program participants was to reduce sedentary time during the day, because any alternative to driving, watching TV, or talking on the phone is likely to generate more steps and be healthier. She found this strategy helped many people get and stay more active, because they found it easier to cut sedentary time than to try to carve out a block of time for exercise. According to Dunn, this substitution strategy can boost your chances of success 10 times.

For an idea of the "substitution" approach, here are eight easy ways to log more steps on your pedometer each day (look for more throughout the book):

1. Get a box at the post office and walk there to pick up your mail.
2. Choose to walk to a more distant cafeteria or deli for lunch. If you brown-bag it, walk to a park or mall and eat there.

PEDOMETER PRO

Is It the Supersize Fries? Or the Lack of Steps?

This is the question most people *don't* ask when they watch the wonderful documentary *Super Size Me*, directed by and starring Morgan Spurlock. But they should! This witty, engaging, and frighteningly educational diary of Spurlock's experiment with eating food *only* from McDonald's for 30 days is a scathing indictment of America's fast-food industry. His shocking weight gain of 24 pounds in just 30 days is only slightly less terrifying than the fact that his doctors said his liver was near collapse by the end of the month, under the pressure of trying to process his fat- and sugar-engorged diet.

Unfortunately, often overlooked but equally compelling are the results of a brief (and we mean brief) cameo by coauthor Mark Fenton, who meets with Spurlock on camera to give him a pedometer and suggest a daily maximum of only 5,000 steps. Mark actually visited at length with Spurlock, who lived in a three-story walk-up in New York City and normally collected 12,000 steps per day. They decided that if Morgan's lifestyle was to truly mimic the disastrous combination of a fast-food diet and life in an automobile-oriented suburb, he should force himself to keep his step total closer to 5,000 a day.

In the movie, Spurlock points out that cab fares alone may bust his budget, as he often has to consciously quit walking by noon in the eminently walkable New York City. But while visiting car-friendly San Antonio, he shows his pedometer topping out at just over 4,000 steps by day's end. (Not surprisingly, there's plenty of research that supports this disheartening anecdote: Where you live appears to have lots to do with how many steps you take.) And although it's impossible to overstate the adverse effects of his fast-food-only diet, there's no doubt that restricting his daily steps only worsened an already unhealthy caloric balance, and vastly diminished his body's ability to handle the extra load.

The good news: After his experiment—and a Sundance Film Festival best director award and Academy Award nomination—Spurlock ate and exercised his way back to health. He admits, however, it took nearly a full year of effort. Maybe his next movie will be *Super Step Me*!

3. Walk to a corner store for newspapers, bread, and milk, even if it costs a bit more.
4. Carpool with a friend and offer to walk all or part of the way to her house for the ride.
5. Skip e-mail—at least occasionally—and hand-deliver messages to coworkers.
6. Walk the kids to school, a friend's house, or the library instead of driving them. (They benefit, too.)
7. Intentionally park at the far end of the parking lot at the mall, grocery store, or office building.
8. Take a quick stroll instead of sitting down for a mid-morning snack.

Keep in mind that it's normal for step counts to ebb and flow somewhat. For example, your total on a Sunday when you relax and catch a football game after a nutty week will be low. But the next Sunday, you might take the family hiking and score an all-time high.

Small Steps to Weight Loss

Can adding steps really help you lose weight? It certainly can. Let's say your weight is currently stable—neither increasing nor decreasing—but you feel that you're 10 pounds overweight. By maintaining your current activities and diet and adding 2,000 steps a day (about 7 miles, or roughly 700 Calories a week), you could lose up to 1 pound every

Make Sure You're Measuring Real Steps

In some cases, pedometers can overcount your steps. This can happen when the device is bumped or jostled, such as while you're riding in a car. Barbara Ainsworth, chair of the Department of Exercise and Nutritional Sciences at San Diego State University, found a way around this when she was studying Native American women. Ainsworth noted unusually high step counts for women who were spending lots of time riding or driving pickup trucks on bumpy dirt roads. To prevent the pedometers from counting at the wrong time, she simply had them open the pedometer case (while still wearing it) so the pedometer could lie flat when traveling in a car or truck. (If your pedometer can't be opened, simply take it off it and lay it flat on the car seat.) Then the device doesn't pick up the vehicle's movement.

If you spend a lot of time in the car, you can do this, too. Of course, for short trips, the additional steps won't throw off your total much and it's probably not worth worrying about. And if you have any doubt, just check your pedometer before and after a ride and note if it's picked up a bunch of steps. Unless you're doing motocross or driving on rough terrain, it's probably not an issue.

five weeks. That's as much as 10 pounds in a year. Although this pace may seem glacial, remember that the weight came on slowly and if you want to lose it for good, it should come off that way, too. After all, the typical American gains one to two pounds a year for most years of adult life—simply reversing that to a modest yearly loss would be a great success.

The proof is in the long-term results. By studying data from a large number of people who had lost 60 pounds and kept it off for five years, researchers at the National Weight Control Registry have shown the success of adding steps. Overall, the successful people ate a low-calorie, low-fat diet (1,380 Calories per day, 20 percent fat—a caloric restriction best made with the guidance of a doctor or nutritionist) and burned 400 Calories per day in exercise. By giving pedometers to a subset of these folks, researchers found that the "successful losers" took an average of 10,900 steps per day. In fact the new U.S. dietary guidelines recommend 60 to 90 minutes of physical activity a day for people who are looking to lose a lot of weight, or to maintain substantial weight loss. Even at a modest 100 steps per minute—a casual pace—that's 6,000 to 9,000 additional steps per day for an otherwise inactive person.

> **STEP BOOSTER**
>
> Climb a flight of stairs in a typical two-story home: 12 to 15 steps per flight. (Do it often.)

The Benefits of More Steps

Weight loss is a goal for countless Americans. But a safe and healthy weight loss program—experts say that losing about a pound every week or two is the smart way to go for permanent success—can seem to take forever. Instead of getting frustrated by this seemingly slow process, try focusing on the many other outcomes that additional walking can bring. Stick with the eventual goal of meeting or exceeding 10,000 steps a day, but know that wherever you're starting, adding smaller increments of steps offers payoffs right away.

How Far Am I Walking, Anyway?

Our approach focuses on adding steps to your day. That's what personalizes it—you know how many steps you started with in Week One, and you can measure your progress against your own baseline.

STEPS TO SUCCESS

The Incremental Benefits of More Steps

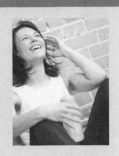

Especially if you're starting at a very low daily step total, know that you can see benefits from even modest increases in your steps. There are no guarantees, given the wide range of individual fitness levels and the intensity of your steps (affected by speed and terrain, for example), but here are some of the benefits of incremental increases in physical activity seen in a wide range of research studies. (The weight loss estimates assume your weight is currently stable; if you're gaining weight now, increasing your steps will likely just slow your rate of weight gain.)

Add This Many Steps per Day	Enjoy These Potential Payoffs
500	Less stress, improved mood
1,200	Modestly reduced risk of heart disease, diabetes, high blood pressure
2,400	Further fortifications of health and mood, increased energy; slow but sustainable weight loss (say, a pound or so every two months)
3,600	Even better health and fitness; more steady weight loss (perhaps 15 pounds a year)
7,200	Dramatically improved health risk and fitness, potential for even faster weight loss (as much as 30 pounds a year)
And what if you walk faster?	
3,000 fast steps	Improved aerobic fitness, boosted HDL (good) cholesterol

PEDOMETER PRO

And Nelly Says It Makes You Feel Good!

At 62, you might guess that Nelly Petrock from Ann Arbor, Michigan, walks to protect her health. She has a family history of high cholesterol, and her readings are now lower, thanks to walking. Her bone density is at the top tenth percentile for her age group, which she attributes to walking and strength training. But her primary reason for walking has little to do with these numbers. She walks to feel good.

"I simply feel so much better when I start the day with 5,000 steps," she says. Her favorite route is a 3-mile jaunt through the nearby University of Michigan campus. On some days, she and her husband drive to another neighborhood to walk, or walk downtown to the bookstore. On rainy days, she puts in 30 minutes on an elliptical trainer at home. When they visit the Netherlands, Nelly's homeland, they walk through ancient towns, past windmills, and along canals.

A mother and grandmother who works at home for her husband's business, Nelly started using a pedometer in 1993. She uses it to gauge her progress toward her daily goal of 10,500 steps. "If I've only done 8,000 steps by dinner, I realize I better get out there and go for a walk," she explains. "It gives me a better mental attitude, knowing that I'm doing something positive for myself."

No standardized miles or kilometers—easier to compile for the fit and speedy, but more challenging for the novice—to confuse the issue or create unrealistic targets.

All well and good, but let's face it—you're still curious about how far you're walking. Maybe you're just charging up the stairs at work, or you've added a nightly stroll with your spouse, or perhaps you're changing your clothes and going out for a full-fledged fitness walk. Whatever it is, you wonder, *How many miles do I walk a day?*

A very simple but rough rule of thumb used by many is 2,000 steps for a mile. It's not a bad average figure, but doesn't account for differences in height, leg and stride length, terrain, and least of all how fast you're walking. After all, as you speed up, your stride naturally lengthens and your steps quicken, but how much depends on your flexibility and fitness level.

Here's the simplest way to estimate your walking distance, and it's as good as any electronic method available. Warm up with several minutes of easy strolling, reset your pedometer to zero,

STEP BOOSTER

Spend an afternoon at the museum of science; ponder the imponderables.

then walk a measured mile, such as four times around a standard quarter-mile high school or college track on the inside lane. The figure you have at the end is your standard "steps per mile" calibration, and don't be surprised by any figure in the 1,600-to-2,400-step range. If you're unsure, simply reset and do it again.

It's important to try to walk at your typical pace—don't get chatting with someone and dawdle (unless that's what you normally do) or get excited and take off like a greyhound. If you tend to walk at different speeds—say, moderate paced for errands or commuting, but speedy when doing "exercise"—then walk a mile at each speed and note the difference in your step total. No doubt the faster mile will require fewer steps because not only are your steps quicker, but your stride has lengthened measurably as well. If you use your pedometer for running, be sure to do a running calibration—your strides will be longer still, and even fewer steps will be needed to cover a mile. Then anytime you walk (or run) at that speed, you can divide the total steps you take by your personal steps-per-mile calibration for an accurate estimate of the distance covered.

Here's an example. Larry walks a measured mile with his pedometer and finds he takes 1,955 steps. Later in the week, he

Exercise Facts

Serving Size	1 mile
Steps Per Mile	About 2000

Amount Per Serving

Calories Burned*	80
Calories from Fat (approx.)	50

	% Daily Value**
Weight Control	**20**%
Blood Pressure Reduction	**21**%
Control of Blood Glucose	**20**%
Cholesterol Improvement	**18**%
Feeling of Vigor	**19**%
Stress Management	**20**%
Cardio-Protection	**20**%

*Calories expended per mile for 150-lb. person (walking at 3 mph).
**Percent daily values are based on a physical activity goal of 10,000 steps per day.

does a walk of 5,073 steps. He divides 5,073 steps by 1,955 steps per mile, to get 5,073 / 1,955 = 2.6 miles.

If your pedometer allows you to input a stride length so that it automatically calculates distance for you, you should still do a full 1-mile calibration walk. Then depending on what the pedometer wants—meters, centimeters, or feet—simply divide 1,609 meters, 160,900 cm, or 5,280 feet by the number of steps you've taken to get a step length you can enter into the device.

Back to Larry, who takes 1,955 steps per mile. To enter his stride length in feet into his pedometer, he divides 5,280 feet by 1,955 steps, to get 2.7 feet per step. If he needed centimeters, he would divide 160,900 centimeters by 1,955 steps, to get 82.3 centimeters per step.

A final note: What if your track only lets joggers on the inner lanes, and relegates walkers to the outer limits? That's fine, but know that you're adding about 3 yards per lap for each lane that you're removed from the inner edge. So if you walk four laps in lane five, you've added about 12 yards a lap, or 48 yards total. Fortunately, the solution is simple: Subtract that distance by stopping early by that amount. In the case of walking in lane five, that's about half the length of the final straightaway (about 50 yards).

A Quick Calorie-Burn Estimate

For a simple estimate of the calories you've burned while walking, do the following calculation. At typical walking speeds of roughly 2 to 4 miles per hour, you can divide your body weight (in pounds) in half to estimate how many calories you burn for each mile of walking.

$$\text{Calories per mile} = \text{Miles Walked} \times \frac{\text{Body Weight (lbs.)}}{2}$$

If you weigh 160 pounds, that's 160 / 2 = 80 Calories per mile. So if you take a 4,500-step walk, you can use the 2,000-step-per-mile rule, and estimate you've walked 2.25 miles. (That's 4,500 steps / 2,000 steps per mile = 2.25 miles.) Your calorie burn estimate is:

2.25 Miles x 80 Calories per Mile = 180 Calories

Of course, not everyone really takes 2,000 steps per mile. To create a more accurate *personal* Calories-per-step equation, do the following onetime calibration:

STEPPING STONE

Small Changes, Big Impact

The evidence that adding a little activity every day is truly effective for better health and weight loss continues to pile up. A Japanese study in 2002, for instance, found that 31 overweight men who added 1,800 steps per day (going from 7,000 to 8,800 steps per day) lost eight pounds in one year. Also impressive: Though the men were told not to make any changes in their eating habits, they tended to consume 100 fewer Calories per day. Proof, perhaps, that one good step leads to another.

Step 1. Walk easily for five minutes to warm up.

Step 2. Walk a measured mile (say, four laps of a one-quarter-mile track) using your pedometer to count how many steps it takes. Typical readings will range from 1,600 to 2,400 steps for a mile. This is your *steps-per-mile* number.

Step 3. Anytime you take a walk, plug the total number of steps you take into the following equation (your body weight must be in pounds):

$$\text{Calories} = \frac{\text{Total Steps Taken}}{\text{Steps per Mile}} \times \frac{\text{Weight (lbs.)}}{2}$$

Example: Cheryl weighs 120 pounds, and has gone to the track and learned she typically takes 2,140 steps per mile. After a long walk, she finds she's taken 7,490 steps. So she calculates:

$$\frac{7{,}490 \text{ Steps}}{2{,}140 \text{ Steps}} \times \frac{120 \text{ (lbs.)}}{2} = 3.5 \text{ Miles} \times \frac{60 \text{ Calories}}{\text{per Mile}} = \frac{210 \text{ Calories}}{\text{per Mile}}$$

Therefore, her walk was about 3.5 miles, and she burned roughly 210 Calories.

Gearing Up for More Steps: Selecting Walking Shoes

As you add more steps, your feet deserve a little attention. After all, heels and dress shoes may look great for work, but they're a pain—literally—even when you're just walking in from the far corner of the parking lot (a perfect way to add steps, by the way). If you're making it a full-fledged walk to the corner store or uptempo jaunt for exercise, having comfortable walking shoes is a must.

The first priority is to get the fit right, so here are tips for trying and buying walking shoes, whatever the style:

- Have both feet measured, and go with the size of the larger foot (they're often a half size or more different).
- Wear the socks you most often wear for walking.
- Try shoes on after noon, when your feet are more swollen to full size.
- Walk around, hop, skip, and dance in the shoes you're trying on. And don't expect them to "break in" and feel better later—if they don't feel great during testing in the store, they certainly won't when you pile on 10,000 steps a day or more.

STEPS TO SUCCESS

Do I Get Credit for Bicycling and Swimming?

They're both great exercise, but you can't use a pedometer in the water, and it will not be accurate on your bike if you're wearing it on your hip. On the bike, clip the pedometer to your shoelaces or sock to measure your pedal revolutions; the reading will be in the ballpark, but not dead accurate. Or you can get around this by using a step equivalent for time in the pool and on the bike. Simply credit yourself with 110 steps for every minute you spend swimming laps or biking—that's a conservative count for a minute of moderately paced walking.

Here's a table you can use to quickly determine how to credit these activities:

Minutes Cycling or Swimming	Steps Earned
15	1,650
20	2,200
30	3,300
45	4,500
60	6,600
90	9,900

The key features to seek in a walking shoe are:

- A very flexible forefoot. Look for the shoe to bend easily where you do, at the ball of your foot.
- A supportive arch. It doesn't have to be built up—choose an arch height based on comfort—but the shoe should *not* bend through the arch. A flimsy arch can lead to soreness, plantar fasciitis (a tightening and chronic inflammation of the sinewy tissue in the sole of your foot), and even heel spurs if worn for too long.
- A rounded or beveled heel. Your foot strikes heel-first when walking, so a low rounded or beveled heel accommodates a smooth heel-to-toe rolling motion. Shoes with built-up or squared-off heels (such as many running or basketball shoes) can lead to shin soreness if you log lots of steps in them.

But what style of walking shoe is right for you? The choices range from a lightweight athletic design—these often look like running shoes but with a more rounded heel—to light hiking

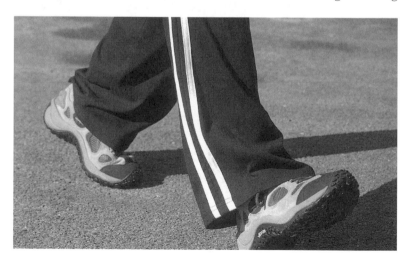

Match Your Shoes to How You Use Them

	Athletic Walking	Dress-Casual	Light Hiking, Rugged Walking
What they offer	Lightweight materials; often breathable synthetics so coolest; super cushioning and flexibility.	More finished appearance; moderate to great cushioning; often midweight range.	Darker, outdoorsy looks; more rugged, thicker outsoles; better traction; more protection on trails and in sloppy weather; can be a bit heavier.
Best for	Faster or more athletic walking; sidewalks, tracks, paved trails, treadmills.	Day-to-day wear, around town, predictable conditions.	From easy to rugged trails and varied terrain; winterwalking.
Be sure to pick if	Cushioning is your greatest need, or speed or fitness is a goal.	You get your steps during the workday, commuting, etc.	You need lots of support; good if you sometimes hike with a pack.

shoes, sometimes called rugged walking shoes, designed for easy to moderate trails. In between lies a range of casual and dress-casual shoes that draw from attributes of each—the lightweight materials of athletic shoes and the support and more finished appearance of hiking shoes. The table above can help you figure out what you might want to try. Whatever style you go with, consider replacing your most used pair every 300 to 500 miles (that's usually three to six months, depending on your typical step totals). Sturdily built hiking shoes may have a slightly longer life span, but know that shoes begin to lose their cushioning and support properties well before they look visibly worn out.

Week Two Program

The good news is that you already know all you need to know. Just keep up your pedometer routine: Wear the pedometer daily, from rising in the morning until you lie down in bed at night. Record your steps for the day, and then reset to zero for the next day.

Plus, you have a new task this week: to boost your daily average by just 20 percent over Week One. Look back at the data from the first week and check your "daily goal for next week." It should show a 20 percent increase. So if you averaged 4,200 steps a day last week, you should have written 5,040 in the daily goal space (4,200 x 1.2). That means this week you're aiming for about 5,000 steps a day.

PEDOMETER PRO

Steve Learns the Cure for Creeping Weight Gain

Steve Burgess, a middle-aged banker from La Crosse, Wisconsin, had steadily gained weight ever since graduating from college. When he hit 262 pounds in 2001, his family doctor advised him to lose weight. What's more, his doc handed him a pedometer and told him to walk 15,000 steps per day to lose weight or 10,000 steps per day to stay at his current weight. Steve liked the idea so much that he began walking immediately. After just one week, he had increased his steps by taking the stairs in his five-story building and including more physical activity throughout his day. Gradually he worked his way up to 15,000 steps, five days a week, and 10,000 steps a day on the other two. Within a year, he had walked off 30 pounds of unhealthy body fat, and he was feeling better than ever. Though Steve also cut calories and watched what he ate, he credits a large part of his success to the pedometer, which motivated him to walk more. In fact, whenever Steve stopped using the pedometer he found the pounds started to creep back on, a reminder that although this is only a six-week program, you may find it beneficial to make wearing a pedometer a long-term habit.

But think of it this way: If you're like lots of Americans, that's only 800 steps more than you were averaging last week, the equivalent of just eight minutes of ambling, or a mere six minutes of brisk, purposeful walking. Plus, you don't have to do it all at once—a minute here, a minute there is fine. Just be sure to get in your additional steps this week, and you'll find how shockingly simple it is to start stepping your way to a longer, healthier life.

Why only boost by 20 percent a week? For two basic reasons. Certainly it's beneficial physiologically. Your body has what scientists call an "adaptive stress response" to exercise. You stress your body by asking it do more than usual (lifting more weight, say, or taking more steps), and it responds by repairing any damage and increasing your capacity to do the work in the future. Muscles get stronger, for example, and you build more capillaries, the small vessels that take blood to the muscle cells. The trick is that your body can only repair and keep up if you do it at a moderate rate, increasing 10 to 20 percent a week. Do lots more, and it can lead to discomfort and even injury.

The second reason has more to do with psychology—the psychology of behavior change. You're going to have to make conscious decisions about how to build more steps into your days, and it won't always be easy. So a gradual approach gives you time to try different things and learn what works and what doesn't.

At the end of the week add up the days for your weekly total, then divide by 7 to determine your daily step average this week. Multiply by 1.2 (a 20 percent increase) and write in your goal for next week. You should already be seeing how you're beginning to incrementally step your way to a healthier, more active lifestyle.

Week Two Step Log

Number of steps	Anything special today?
Monday	
Tuesday	
Wednesday	
Thursday	
Friday	
Saturday	
Sunday	
Week Total	

Daily average: _____
(total steps for the week divided by 7)

Daily goal for next week: _____
(daily average x 1.2, for a 20% increase)

Week Three

*Walking Toward the Gold Standard
of 10,000 Steps a Day*

You've got the groove, so now it's time to build up the steps. The first two weeks were easy—in Week One you just measured your baseline, and in Week Two you were excited to see how fast the steps piled up. *Hey, I just went to the mailbox . . . and got 72 steps!* This week the goal is to build some of those modest step increases into permanent additions and to make your newer steps into habits. More important, it's time to begin looking toward a larger goal: 10,000 steps or more.

How Many Steps Are Enough?

The answer, of course, depends on your personal desires, but 10,000 steps per day is a widely accepted recommendation among health and fitness experts. Many believe that getting "10K a day" (as in 10,000 steps, not 10 kilometers) is roughly equivalent to the surgeon general's recommendation to include a minimum of 30 minutes of moderate activity—such as walking—every day. But where did this nice round number come from?

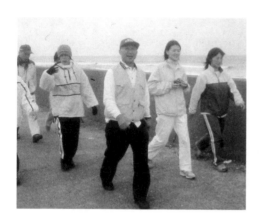

On the heels of the Tokyo Olympics in 1964, the Japanese realized that while elite athletes were in fine shape, little was being done to promote exercise for the rest of the population. Experts made an educated guess for a healthy goal, and tied it to the catchy slogan, "10,000 steps per day."

Through the years, this benchmark has been supported by more and more evidence. In 1975, Japanese researcher Dr. Yoshiro Hatano showed that 10,000 steps a day requires at least 333 Calories of energy expenditure for an average-sized Japanese person. This was significant, because it was roughly the same amount of exercise that experts were concluding gives protection from heart

STEPPING STONE

The Japanese Have a Word for It

In Japan, the word for pedometer is *manpo-kei*, which, translated literally, means "ten thousand steps meter."

PEDOMETER PRO

Yoshiro Hatano: Pedometer Pioneer

You could call researcher Dr. Yoshiro Hatano from Miyazaki, Japan, the father of 10,000 steps. After all, he's been studying pedometers and the benefits of walking since the 1965 launch of the Japanese "10,000 steps a day" slogan that was designed to encourage activity among its citizens. One of his most significant findings was that 10,000 steps a day burned about the same amount of calories that health experts recommend for protection against heart attacks and strokes. Some of his most recent research has centered on older people, and he found that regular walkers suffered far fewer health problems such as hypertension, diabetes, coronary heart disease, and mental stress than nonwalkers of the same age. Beyond good health, these seniors reported fulfillment, engagement with cultural hobbies, sound sleep, strong immunity, and freedom from becoming "TV maniacs."

Hatano practices what he preaches. He wears a pedometer every day, and has been loyal to the slogan he's worked to support. From 1980 to 1998, he averaged 12,800 steps per day. Since moving from Tokyo to a more rural setting and finding more leisure time for walking, he has averaged 14,000 steps per day.

attacks and strokes. In the landmark College Alumni Study—a classic because of its size and scope—Dr. Ralph Paffenbarger surveyed 17,000 men to determine their physical activity habits, and then followed up with them 6 to 10 years later. He observed that alumni who burned 300 Calories per day through walking, stair climbing, and leisure-time physical activity had half as many heart attacks as their sedentary peers. This protective effect of an active lifestyle has been confirmed by numerous large-scale studies of both men and women since the 1970s.

Additional studies have shown that people who are regularly active—particularly in bouts of 10 minutes or more—stack the

STEPPING STONE

Five Reasons Why the 10,000-Steps-a-Day Goal Works

1. It's a concrete goal. And a pedometer provides immediate feedback on whether you're meeting it.
2. It focuses on a daily behavior that's under your control, not an elusive goal, like "to lose weight." The needle on the bathroom scale never seems to move; your pedometer count moves with every step.
3. It's one size fits all. Because this goal is expressed in steps, not calories, it doesn't depend on body weight. So even if you lose weight, the target remains the same.
4. It brings freedom of choice. A 20-year-old might get her steps by playing soccer and trail running, a 45-year-old might play tennis and walk with coworkers at lunch, and a 75-year-old might walk at a local mall or indoor track or during volunteer work.
5. It counts activity throughout the day. Previously, experts focused on exercise as separate from "real life," without considering occupation, mode of transportation, or the intensity of daily routine.

deck in their favor for good health. Some of these findings indicate that:

- Japanese people who take 10,000 steps per day have lower blood pressure and less body fat than those who walk less.
- Sedentary, at-risk people who start logging 10,000 steps per day record improvements in body weight, blood pressure, and glucose tolerance.
- You can cut your risk of heart disease equally with either one bigger chunk—say, 30 minutes—or several shorter

bouts of exercise, according to Harvard researcher Dr. I-Min Lee.

Because it is possible to log 10,000 steps a day with light, intermittent physical activity, experts at the Centers for Disease Control point out that it's uncertain that the 10,000-steps-a-day goal ensures adequate intensity to protect against heart disease. However, our experience suggests that sedentary people who normally take 5,000 steps or fewer per day almost always need to add one to three conscious and continuous bouts of activity (totaling 30 to 50 minutes) to their day to reach a goal of 10,000 steps. So taking 10,000 steps a day may not *guarantee* that you'll meet the national physical activity recommendations, but it makes it much more *likely* that you'll hit the minimum recommendation of 30 minutes of moderate physical activity.

> **STEP BOOSTER**
> Walk down the street to visit a neighbor.

Targeting *Your* Magic Number

With a look at the sedentary nature of much of American life, you might conclude it's time to dump modern conveniences and go no-tech, like the Amish. In fact, coauthor David Bassett has studied this lifestyle in depth, and thinks it might not be a bad idea. He found that Amish people living in a traditional farming community in Ontario get plenty of activity—most sit for an average of three hours a day (compared with our typical eight to 10), and are active for roughly 50 hours per week, with a good bit of strenuous work thrown in for good measure. Daily step totals averaged around 14,200 for women and 18,400 for men. One man hit 51,500 steps in a day, and one woman got in 10,000 steps before

STEPPING STONE

Why Are the Amish So Active?

The Amish people are a Protestant group who originated in Switzerland but came to North America beginning around 1727. Though we can't do justice to their full system of beliefs here, it's notable that at their core the Amish value simplicity, nonviolence, and traditional values, as opposed to the current vogue, which focuses on progress and technology. Farming is the most common occupation, and Amish men till the soil with horses and harvest crops without tractors. Amish women do most of the child care, vegetable gardening, and an array of chores from cooking and canning to making, cleaning, and mending clothes and household items. Given that they don't own cars, walking and horse-drawn carriages are their primary transportation modes, and with no electricity or telephones in their homes, sedentary entertainments such as television and surfing the Web certainly aren't options. Not that the Amish have a lot of time left over for such inactive pursuits, anyway.

breakfast! Despite their hearty diets of meat, potatoes, vegetables, and desserts, there is little obesity among this particular study group. This suggests that by eating a moderate diet, you can pursue a more moderate step goal and still stay in balance (and you might even get to keep your cell phone).

Clearly, all the variables in the mix make it impossible to come up with a one-size-fits-all magic number. The right goal for you depends on your physiology, how much and what you eat, and how fast you walk. Say you walk 12,000 steps a day and want to lose weight, but you won't give up your ice cream or trade double-cheese pepperoni pizza for plain cheese. You'll need to add even more steps. Or maybe you're happy with your weight but you'd really like to be able to gallop up those two flights from the subway or keep up with your kids without gasping for breath. You may only need

8,000 steps a day, but you'd better take 5,000 of them quickly enough to boost your heart rate and get you to break a sweat.

The Big Picture on Steps

Here's a quick look at the number of steps you might shoot for each day, based on what you hope to achieve over the long run. And here's some comforting news: Although we're focusing on daily step totals, you may find it easier to think in terms of a weekly target. That's especially true if your schedule invariably makes some days (say, when you spend lots of time in the car) worse than others for collecting steps. So use the daily goals as a target, but don't panic if you have variation from day to day throughout the week. In the end, hitting your weekly total is just as beneficial.

For starters, the goal should simply be to increase your daily activity level by adding steps. But your eventual step target depends on your aspirations. Here are three basic targets to shoot for:

Daily Step Totals for Healthy Adults

Your Personal Goal	Average Daily Step Target
Reduced risk for chronic illness (such as heart disease, diabetes, cancer) and moderate weight loss.	At least 10,000 steps/day (70,000 steps/week)
Long-term health, plus more noticeable weight loss (the higher you go, the faster the pounds come off)	12,000–15,000 steps/day (84,000–105,000 steps/week)
Increased aerobic fitness (heart and lung strength)	At least 10,000 steps per *week* at a *fast* pace (enough to create noticeable breathing and a boosted heart rate)*

*Note: Spread these faster steps over at least three days of the week in chunks of 3,000 steps or more.

Is 10,000 Steps Right for All Ages?

Though 10,000 is a perfectly memorable number and easy to focus on as you check your pedometer throughout the day, it's probably not the right target for absolutely everyone. Certainly anyone looking for a more rapid rate of weight loss will benefit from more daily steps, and frankly if you're currently gaining weight and are

 STEPPING STONE

Stepping Across the Ages

The sad truth: Not only are American adults inactive, but so are our children, as is revealed by a look at step-count averages from elementary-school-aged kids from the American Southwest compared with those of children around the world. But it gets worse. The only reason American children appear to be so close to their Australian peers is that swimming—a superpopular activity in Australia that provides lots of exercise for their children—doesn't register in step counts. This suggests that American children are even farther behind. In addition to being less active, the studies that collected body-weight data suggest American children are more overweight, too. Equally disconcerting is the trend for girls to be less active than boys, likely a result of social norms more than any physiological factors.

Country	Average Step Count	Boys	Girls
Belgium	15,038	16,600	13,000
Sweden	14,900	16,200	13,600
United Kingdom	14,000	16,000	12,700
Australia	13,000	14,300	11,700
United States	12,000	13,200	11,000

There's a similar dearth of data for older adults. Not surprisingly, step totals do seem to decline with age, but that begs the big question: What's the cause and what's the effect? Many of us can name some spry 70-year-a really big eater (and don't plan on changing that), you may need more than 10,000 steps just to get your weight to stabilize. On the other hand, if you have an injury or chronic illness, 10,000 or even 7,000 steps may be unrealistically high as a minimum target. Talk to your doctor about what's right for you. But what about older or younger people?

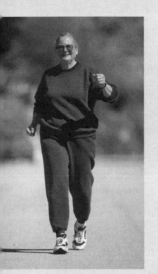

old who seems incessantly active and possessed of an endless supply of energy. Now, that could in part be due to great genetics. But it's also likely a result of having remained active through age 70! To dramatically reduce step recommendations for older adults may be creating a self-fulfilling prophecy—if you become less active, you're less fit and healthy, and it follows that you're inclined to be less active. Another step in what can be a debilitating cycle of aging. Therefore, if you're healthy and your doctor agrees, you should probably stick with the 10,000-step-per-day minimum for as long as you can. That said, our observations suggest it's common to see the step averages drop somewhat as people move into their 70s, 80s, and beyond. So be realistic while working to remain active.

A final point—this all assumes you're in good health, without metabolic or musculoskeletal problems that would challenge your ability to accumulate steps. People with chronic illnesses or physical limitations may find that 10,000 or even 7,000 steps per day simply isn't realistic. In that case, the best thing to do is to discuss your situation with your health care professional, and to set a goal that is realistic and health inducing, not angst producing. After all, adding steps should be not only physically attainable and healthful, but also emotionally rewarding and fun.

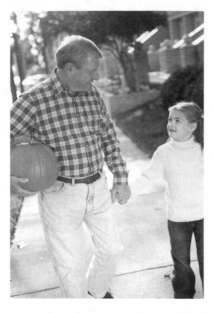

Unfortunately, there are not yet reams of data on step counting in children or in older adults. Based on the small amount of average data available on American kids, the President's Council on Physical Fitness and Sports has set the following minimums for children shooting to earn their Active Lifestyle Award: boys 13,000 steps per day; girls, 11,000. Though that's not a bad start, it has two major limitations.

First, it's based only on *current* average step totals. Yet with American youth showing early signs of the obesity epidemic that's plaguing American adults, it's very possible that children's current levels of physical activity are anything but sufficient, especially given the typical diet of an American youngster. Further, note that U.S. kids lag behind their international peers (see "Stepping Stone: Stepping Across the Ages" on page 48), and are generally heavier than more active kids in other countries.

STEP BOOSTER

Give the kids more steps; assign them physically active, age-appropriate chores.

Second, the lower step recommendation for girls may be the sad reflection of a culture that undervalues physical activity or athleticism in young women. After all, we don't give *adult* women a lower recommendation than adult men. So by no means be satisfied by the targets of 13,000 steps for boys and 11,000 steps for girls—consider them a minimum starting point, while encouraging your kids to be as active as possible.

STEPPING STONE

Walking Around the World

It seems that American adults take fewer steps than those in other countries. Of course, these are only small samples, but they are averages representative of their regions. And the good news is that there are countries where the average is very close to 10,000 steps per day. If they can do it, so can you!

Country	Steps per Day	Number of Adults Tested
Switzerland	9,700	493
Western Australia	9,695	428
Japan	8,200	500
U.S. (Colorado)	6,804	742
U.S. (South Carolina)	5,931	209

10,000 Steps and Weight Loss—It Can Happen

An encouraging study in 2005 by Patrick Schneider, PhD, an assistant professor in the Human Performance Laboratory at Ball State University in Indiana, suggests that if you're overweight and inactive, a 10,000-step-per-day routine can lead to modest but meaningful weight loss. At the outset, Schneider measured the height, weight, body fat, blood pressure, and blood lipid profile of 56 people. He also had them record their steps for one week (they averaged 5,100 steps per day). They were then instructed to gradually increase until they were taking 10,000 steps per day. They recorded their daily steps on a log sheet, and at the end of each week they turned in their logs and averages were calculated. Does this sound remotely familiar?

After nine months, the participants returned for follow-up measurements. Schneider found that people who faithfully adhered to the 10,000-step-per-day recommendation lost nearly 10

STEPS TO SUCCESS

Your Pedometer as a *Speedometer*

The faster your walk, the longer *and faster* your steps will be. This comes in handy not only when you're bolting to catch the bus, but also when you're trying to squeeze in more steps in less time. You can even roughly gauge your speed by knowing how many steps you take in just 20 seconds. Simply glance at your watch and count your steps for 20 seconds (or let your pedometer do the work for a full minute to be more accurate), then look up your count below for the corresponding speed. For more detailed information on estimating your walking speed, see Week Five.

Walking Speeds at Various Step Rates

Steps Taken in 20 Sec.	Steps per Minute	Estimated Speed (mph)	How Does It Feel?
33	100	2.0–2.5	Dawdling, ambling, chatting
40	120	3.0–3.5	Purposeful but easy walking (a healthy pace)
45	135	3.5–4.0	Focused, brisk walking (a calorie-burning tempo)
50	150	4.0–4.5	Aerobic-fitness-building speed; bent arms and quick steps
55	165	4.5–5.0	Fast aerobic walking; beginning racewalking
60	180	5.5–6.0+	Fast racewalking; jogging
65	195	6.5+	Competitive racewalking; running

pounds by the end of the study. Not surprisingly, those who hadn't increased their step totals saw little or no change in their body weight. In short, he found that you've got to stick with it to see results. And to be clear, we're not suggesting this is an opportunity to use a 5,000-step walk as an excuse to eat an extra doughnut, just because they both equal about 240 Calories. Fortunately, many people find that as they become more active, they are inclined to eat more healthfully—it seems they don't want to regain through bad diet what they've worked so hard to lose through activity.

Now, 10 pounds in nine months is barely more than a pound a month. But keep in mind that's an average for those who adhered

STEP BOOSTER

Move your washer and dryer to the basement: 120 steps for every two loads of laundry.

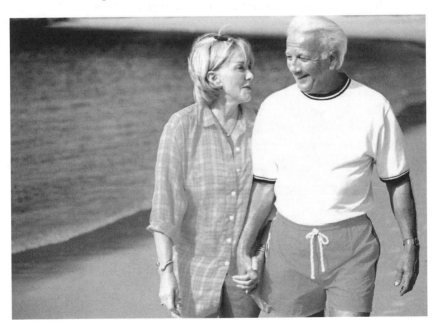

to the program, and it doesn't take into account what they were doing with their diets. One man who lost 22 pounds spoke proudly of his "belt of honor." As time passed and the pounds melted away, he had to punch new holes in his belt to make it smaller. Another woman was overjoyed because she had lost enough weight so that she was no longer classified as clinically obese (30 to 40 pounds overweight for a woman of average height).

When asked to summarize his study, Schneider quipped, "10,000 steps for man, one giant leap for mankind!" Pretty snappy for a research guy, don't you think? And very encouraging news for anyone looking to make permanent progress toward a healthier weight.

Eliminate Your Top Step Stealers

Adding steps to your day is a great way to move closer to greater health and gain energy. But another way to make progress is to eliminate (or at least reduce) the amount of time you spend in energy-sapping, calorie-hoarding, physically *inactive* pursuits.

How to Make Walking Part of Your Life, Every Day

1. Walk every day. Try to stick to the schedule that we lay out in the program, but if you can only get out for 5 or 10 minutes, it's better than nothing.
2. Record it. Write down your step total every day. If you did a specific, continuous walk, note how far or how long it was, too.
3. Be flexible. There will be times when you have to swap the schedule around to make sure you get your steps in. Make

Lose Your Top Step Stealers

Don't let these culprits make off with your valuable time and steps. Here's how to foil them:

Instead of	Try to gain	Think about
Multiple short car trips per day.	2,400 steps (two swift 10-minute errands on foot).	Ten trips a day isn't uncommon for a typical suburban household; make some into walks or bike rides.
One large car trip per day.	5,000 steps (~2.5 miles, less than an hour).	The average American commuter spends 24.3 minutes a day in the car. That's more than 100 hours a year on your rear.
Turning on the TV.	7,000 steps for 60 minutes.	Americans typically veg out for more than four hours of television per day; make at least one hour a brisk walk instead of a lazy "watch."
Passive socializing.	1,200 steps for 10 minutes.	Turn 10 minutes of yakking at the office coffee station or school pickup into 10 minutes of talk-while-you-walk.
E-mail correspondence.	600 steps to a neighbor or nearby office.	Sometimes it's a real time-saver, but do you really need to e-mail your neighbor for that recipe? Walk over and ask her instead.
Video games.	1,950 steps of *real* games.	Replace 15 minutes with any active game outdoors, from hopscotch to hoops.
Web surfing.	3,000 steps (30 minutes) of actual, not virtual, shopping.	The World Wide Web is an information miracle, but a disaster for human activity levels now that we can shop, research, and be entertained all while we sit on our tailbones.

it work for you. Take longer walks when you have more time, and work in shorter bouts on busier days.

4. Spread out the big-total days. Avoid getting to Thursday and noticing that your count is too low for the week. Bunching together several higher-than-normal step-count days can be hard on your body and your schedule. Spread them out for variety and rest.

5. Listen to your body. If you're feeling tired or sore from walking, take it down a notch. If you're not challenged, try skipping to the next week's prescription.

6. Walk every day. Yes, we said that already. But it bears repeating. Break walks into 10-minute mini-walks if it helps, and look for other ways to be active each day.

 STEPS TO SUCCESS

Pedometers Can Help Everyone

If you belong to an ethnic group with higher obesity rates, is 10,000 steps still enough? Some researchers questioned this, too, and found the answer to be yes, at least in part. A study conducted in 2003 by Dr. Melicia Whitt, PhD, and colleagues at the University of Pennsylvania School of Medicine looked at step rates for African American women, who have an obesity rate of nearly 50 percent, compared with 31 percent for other American adults. By measuring and comparing steps taken per day, Whitt found that healthy-weight African American women took an average of 9,997 steps per day, while overweight women took 7,595 steps per day, and obese women took an average of 6,210 steps per day. These numbers suggest that 10,000 steps a day is a fitting goal—or at least a good initial target—for African American women to reach healthy weights, too.

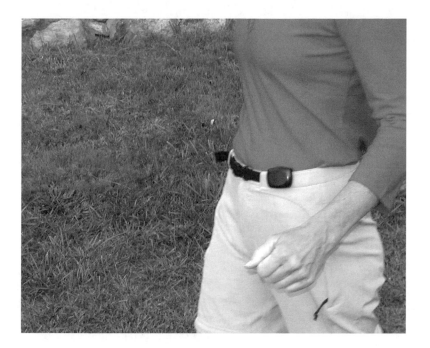

Week Three Program

No doubt you've gotten the routine down now: putting on your pedometer first thing in the morning, taking the pedometer off at the end of the day, writing down your steps, and resetting the pedometer to zero. You're also already getting a sense of what tends to add steps to your day, and what tends to take them away. You may even recognize a weekly pattern evolving. Some people find weekends more active, thanks to chores and recreation; others find that's when they kick back to relax. If you haven't already, this is a good week to start looking at your pedometer throughout the day. Of course, you don't want to be a head case about it. ("Oh, my gosh! It's noon and I'm only at 3,200 steps. Better skip that

Kathy Finds an Extra Short Walk Does the Trick

Kathy Riordan, a former college basketball star who once scored 49 points in a game, scores more steps than hoops these days. A 60-year-old office manager from Knoxville, Tennessee, Kathy learned about pedometers when she volunteered for a study at the University of Tennessee. Two years later and eight pounds lighter, she's still wearing hers.

Her office building is almost the size of a football field, and although she walks as much as she can at work, Kathy says that this alone is not enough. But if she changes shoes to team up with a coworker or two and walks briskly around the company grounds at lunch, she gets a good workout in about 30 minutes. Adding this 3,000-plus-step walk means she can usually hit 10,000 steps by the end of the day. On other days, she walks at home after work with her husband for 30 minutes around their neighborhood, and gets nearly 4,000 steps. They also take longer, 90-minute walks on trails and in parks. "I like the socialization aspect, and it's a lot easier with a buddy," she says. "And I have more energy when I exercise."

kidney transplant I had scheduled and head out for a walk instead.") But you'll find keeping tabs on your progress can keep you marching toward your goal all day, and not always hustling for another 2,000 steps at 9:00 PM. (Unless, of course, that's when you like to go for a walk.)

Assuming you're not yet at the 10,000-step-per-day level, average your daily totals from Week Two, then boost the daily goal for Week Three by 20 percent again. If the 20 percent jumps are too challenging, back it down to a 10 percent boost, or just hold your step levels steady for a week or two while your new level of activity becomes a habit. But don't lose sight of eventually building up to at least the 10,000-step-per-day minimum.

If, on the other hand, you're already at the 10,000 step level, you can simply try to maintain that and see how it feels. However, if losing substantial weight is a serious goal, don't necessarily be content at 10,000 a day. That's a great start, but if you're insistent on losing pounds more quickly, you should consider targeting 12,000 steps a day or more. And if weight loss is really your focus, don't underestimate the importance of a balanced, moderate diet to your long-term success. That said, 10,000 steps is a great minimum target, with the benefits only likely to be greater at higher step totals.

A final thought: It's fine to start thinking about your weekly as well as daily goal now. You'll find it especially helpful during a week when you have an unusually low day—say, you stayed late at work, or had all-afternoon chauffeur duty for the kids. By adding steps on two or three other days, you can still hit your goal for the week, and thus maintain your *average* daily steps.

Week Three Step Log

Number of steps	Anything special today?
Monday	
Tuesday	
Wednesday	
Thursday	
Friday	
Saturday	
Sunday	
Week Total	

Daily average: _____
(total steps for the week divided by 7)

Daily goal for next week: _____
(daily average x 1.2, for a 20% increase)

Week Four

Hiking Up Your Step Total

Now the race is on. You've probably found the easy-to-add steps buried under your busy lifestyle. The real question is whether you can find those clever, and perhaps a bit more challenging, ways to add activity to your days. The trick now may be to make it a more conscious effort—deciding to leave the car behind even when it means you've got to remember your knapsack and shopping list so you can pick up groceries on the way home, or getting up a bit earlier for a brisk walk before getting the kids off to school. This week we want to suggest that merely going out for a walk can be one of the most simple and effective ways to add steps. Follow our advice and you'll find it's one of the most fun, too.

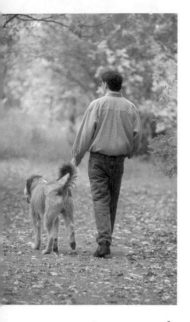

Adding Walks to Your Week

Given your increasing step targets, simply building extra steps here and there throughout the week may not be enough. You're likely off to a good start and have a much greater awareness of how active or sedentary you are, and hopefully you've peeled away some of those more lethargic habits (two hours of TV a night) and replaced them with more energetic options (an after-dinner "constitutional" with the dog). But how do you keep adding 20 percent to your daily step goal?

One approach is to add longer chunks of activity. This is particularly helpful in light of the fact that the overall goal is to average a certain amount of activity over the week. Here's the rub: If you have several busy days when your step counts are lower (and we all do), you'll need to work in some conscious, longer walks to make up for it. Here are three great ways to do it that are not only fairly easy, but actually enjoyable as well:

1. Join or start a walking group or club.
2. Sign up and train for a walking (or running) event.
3. Plan and prepare for a half-day or longer hike.

The Gang's All Here

Walking is by far the most popular physical activity in America, and clubs and groups are sprouting up like weeds. They range from fun to formal, from casual to competitive. And they are offshoots

PEDOMETER PRO

Laura Makes It Stick by Making It Social

As a labor and delivery nurse, 43-year-old Laura Bassett from Knoxville, Tennessee, spends plenty of time on her feet. By wearing a pedometer for a year to track her steps, she found that she averaged 11,740 steps per day on working days. To make sure she gets enough exercise on days when she's not on duty, Laura walks regularly. A social person who prefers to visit with others when she's exercising, she and five friends started the Lunch Bunch. When all of their children were young, the moms split into groups; one group took care of the kids while the others walked; then they swapped. Fourteen years later, all of their children are now in school, but the women still meet for 3-mile walks and lunch.

of a surprisingly wide variety of organizations and entities. Here's a quick list of places to look for a walking group in your area. If they don't have one already, many would love to host a group of walkers if you're willing to simply take the lead:

- Health and fitness clubs, YMCAs. Outdoor walking programs are increasingly common in centers that used to focus on classes and indoor exercise.
- Hospitals, HMOs, clinics, wellness and rehabilitation centers. Walking is the favorite activity for cardiac rehab, but more and more health programs see the value of promoting walking to prevent costly diseases such as diabetes. Your health insurance might even underwrite participation in such a program.
- Parks and recreation departments. Many use their trails and facilities as the basis for innovative walking programs, sometimes combining walking and environmental education.

STEPS TO SUCCESS

Subsidize Your Walking Group

Here's a nutty idea: While walking, keep an eye out for valuables along the road. Okay, this really won't help a club get going, but four-time Olympic racewalker Carl Schueler has accumulated almost an entire metric socket set from the roadside, and figures he can send his daughter to college on collected spare change thanks to his eagle eye. (Well, almost.) Maybe you can help underwrite the club picnic with what you find.

- Worksites. Employers love to have more active employees—research shows they're more productive, healthier, and absent less often—and many companies launch formal wellness programs utilizing pedometers.
- Conservation and land protection groups. Many see sharing and exploring natural areas as a way to help more people value these special places and help protect them.
- Senior centers and community centers. Increasingly, senior-oriented programs focus on helping aging Americans to maintain physically active and thus independent lifestyles.

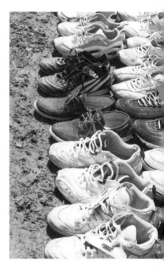

- Historical societies, garden clubs. Community groups often recognize that the best way to share their assets, from historical properties to showcase gardens, is with walking tours. Be a docent and see how many steps you log!
- Neighborhood associations, book clubs—anything else you can imagine.

In fact, any group that convenes to talk can convene to walk—and might find they get a lot more done that way, too!

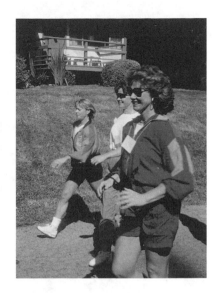

If you decide to get a walking group together, don't set yourself up for failure by making it too complicated. Focus on a few simple things to get started:

- Set a time and place where you'll meet regularly to walk, and don't let the weather deter you. Get in the habit of walking rain or shine; whoever can make it, will. If possible, collect e-mail addresses; it makes communicating with the group especially easy.
- Don't spend a lot of time worrying about making rules and paying dues. Some of the most successful groups have the least structure. An occasional group social outing (say, a postwalk breakfast on Saturday morning) and pitching in for group T-shirts or hats (invariably an opportunity for great artistic creativity) may be all you need.
- Encourage members to walk in groups of similar ability and fitness. Speedsters may feel frustrated if they are stuck with a group of chatters; a beginner may get turned off if dropped in with a bunch of fitness fanatics.

The real key, of course is to have fun. Getting out with people of like mind and making it a regular habit are all it really takes.

Ready, Set, Go!

Signing up for an event can provide a double boost to your step totals—the walk itself is a great step accumulator, but even more valuable is the incentive it provides ahead of time. As you walk to

STEPPING STONE

America's Number One Exercise

Walking is the nation's most popular form of exercise, according to a survey by the U.S. National Center for Health Statistics. The table below lists the percentage of American adults who reported doing each activity in a previous two-week period. And though walking is tops, it's certainly not your only option; even if you're not an avid walker, your pedometer will record most of these activities (with the exception of swimming and water sports). Bicycling is a bit of a challenge, but if you clip the pedometer to your sock or shoelaces it gives a fairly accurate indication of your pedal strokes, which is a fine way to get credit for another great physical activity.

How Active Are America's Favorite Activities?

Activity	Popularity (% of Adults Participating)	Typical Calories Burned in 30 Min.	Typical Steps 30 Min.
Walking, moderate pace	44.1	136	3,467
Walking, brisk pace	(incl. above)	180	4,050
Yard work (e.g., mowing)	29.4	186	2,910
Stretching exercises (e.g., yoga)	25.5	85	96
Bicycling (or stationary bike)	15.4	204	2,877
Weight lifting or other exercises	14.1	205	402
Stair climbing	10.8	330	2,800
Running, moderate pace	9.1	341	4,725

get in shape for a 5- or 10-kilometer walk (and you should), you'll be piling on the steps.

There's a growing array of walking events to choose from, from 1-mile "fun walks" at running races to formal 50-kilometer (that's

Activity	Popularity (% of Adults Participating)	Typical Calories Burned in 30 Min.	Typical Steps 30 Min.
Aerobics	7.1	290	2,564
Swimming for exercise	6.5	306	0
Tennis	2.7	239	2,276
Bowling	4.1	102	651
Golf	4.9	102	956
Baseball or softball	3.5	171	1,192
Handball, racquetball, or squash	1.6	239	2,018
Cross-country skiing	0.4	396	3,006
Basketball	5.8	282	2,730
Soccer	0.9	239	2,493
Other activities, including:	5.7		
Badminton		153	1,326
Dancing (fox-trot)		102	1,233
Figure skating		188	584
Tai chi		136	100

Most of the step counts and calorie estimates come from researcher Jenny Oliver, who had 287 students at the University of Tennessee wear pedometers during a variety of activities. Her findings bear out that some sports, such as figure skating and weight training, don't require a lot of steps even though they burn many calories. But by and large, the more strenuous activities require more steps than the less vigorous ones, just as you'd expect.

about 31 miles) competitions. So here's a summary to help you pick the distance that's right for you.

First-Timers — 1 Mile to 5 Kilometers (3.1 Miles)

Short walks are perfect if you've never walked an event before because they don't require too much training, and you get a taste of details such as sign-ups and self-pacing without risk of serious problems. These are ideal if you average 5,000 to 8,000 steps a day. A 5-kilometer is also great if you're working on boosting your speed and want a short, speedy effort.

The 5 and 10 Range — 5 Miles to 10 Kilometers (6.2 Miles)

These are very common distances, and anyone who can walk 75 to 90 minutes with relative ease should have no problem. Many running races that also feature associated walks are this long, making them great events to test your fitness—there will certainly be other folks walking at or near your speed. Plus, many have great food and prizes afterward!

Endurance Tests — 10 Miles to Half-Marathon (13.1 Miles)

There's a half-day commitment needed for 10-mile or longer walks, and a commitment needed to train for them, too. However, they're still short enough that you can prepare with occasional longer walks (of two hours or 14,000 steps or more) plus a couple of shorter but faster walks each week. Save this distance until you're a committed six-day-a-week walker who can walk two and a half hours at a stretch, and you've got at least two or three

STEP BOOSTER

Sign up for a charity walk and bring along a friend. Train ahead of time.

solid months of walking at this level under
your belt.

The Long Haul — 20 Miles, Marathon (26.2 Miles), and 50 Kilometers (31 Miles)

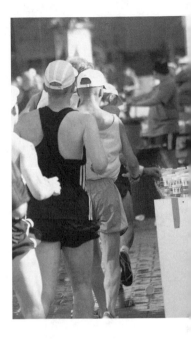

Not as wacky as you might think, fund-raising
groups such as the Leukemia Society and
Arthritis Foundation train hundreds of regular
walkers a year to successfully walk a marathon
—easily 48,000 steps or more. And these can
be tremendously rewarding events, but they
also require the most demanding preparation.
Only tackle a marathon if you're walking daily,
have committed yourself to several challenging workouts a week for four months or more,
and have built up to four and a half hours or more in your longest
weekly efforts. That may not get you a blazing-fast time, but it will
be enough to get you through a marathon safely and respectably.

Ultra-Events — 50 Miles and Beyond

Yes, there really are walking events this long. A 50-miler could
take 100,000 steps and more than 12 hours to complete, while
some racewalkers aspire to the ultimate challenge of becoming a
"centurion," walking 100 miles in under 24 hours. (There are also
multiday long-distance walks that are less daunting.) But don't
even think about these unless you're completely committed to
serious training for six months or more—and even then, know
that events this long can leave well-prepared athletes entirely
wiped out. The flip side? A walk this long is an extraordinary
accomplishment, and training for it will likely get you in the best

STEPS TO SUCCESS

What Type of Event Should I Do?

Not sure what kind of event you're ready to try? Let this table help you sort through the options.

Type of Event	Great For	But Watch Out
Volksmarches. Usually 10K (6.2 miles), on a marked course, with open start times.	Noncompetitive, go-as-you-please types looking to get in their miles.	Very low-key, and courses range from the striking to the mundane. Check ahead online.
Fund-raisers. Usually heavily sponsored, formal events, from 1 to 60 miles (for multiday walks).	Those who want to support a cause and walk with lots of like-minded folks. Usually prizes and goodie bags are offered.	A specific and even substantial donation may be required, and the cause may pervade the event.
Fitness and health promotions. Often hospital/HMO sponsored, 5K to 10K typical (3.1 to 6.2 miles).	Anyone looking for lots of information and inspiration to lead a healthier lifestyle.	May be preachy—how much more do you want to hear about heart disease?
Running races. Most road races now have formal or informal walking divisions.	Folks hoping to walk fast and do their best on an accurately measured course that will be a good test of fitness.	Walkers can be treated as second-class citizens, starting later and getting left out of prize drawings—check the entry form to be sure.
Racewalks. Organized by local clubs, most events feature a wide range of race-walkers, from novices and seniors to serious competitors.	Anyone seeking racewalk instruction; you'll be swept up by this fraternal, dedicated, and often off-the-wall group of athletes.	The technique is challenging, and in real events the judges can disqualify (DQ) you; still, novices are treated warmly, and often are given only instruction, not DQs.

shape of your life. Try to get a few marathons under your belt before pondering an ultra-distance event.

Hit the Trail

Want all the fun of accumulating steps, a boost in fitness benefits, a change of scenery, and maybe a bit of adventure, too? If so, then it's time to head out for a hike. A longer weekend hike can really boost your weekly step total, but even a midweek amble on nearby conservation land can provide a fresh setting, new challenge, and welcome change from your weekday routines. Plus, by its nature hiking is more social, affording the opportunity to spend (dare we say it?) quality time with friends and family.

If you're at a loss for how to choose a hike, check with the hiking groups listed in the Resources section at the end of this book.

Even if you're not near a mountain, chances are there's a nature preserve or trail system close to you. For other suggestions, talk with friends, outdoor store staffers, and guidebooks. As you mull over your options, think about what might motivate you. After all, choosing a destination with a payoff, such as a summit, lookout point, or waterfall, can be half the fun.

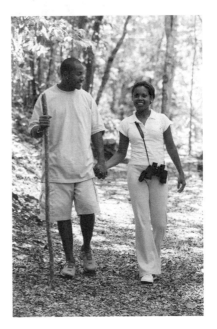

Wherever you go, here are a few principles that will help keep a hike enjoyable, and leave you enthused to come and do it again. And after all, isn't that what it's all about?

PEDOMETER PRO

Encounter with a Living Fountain of Youth

During a 13-mile hike up Mount Cammerer in Great Smoky Mountains National Park, coauthor David Bassett met a spry 68-year-old man from Pennsylvania. They hiked and talked on the way down from the stone lookout tower at the summit, and the older man explained how getting more active had changed the quality of his life. Shortly before retiring, he had had a complete physical exam, including a treadmill test, and the results were about average for someone his age.

Two years later, after stepping up his walking, he took another treadmill test. His doctor was astonished to see him tirelessly attack a steep grade on the treadmill without breaking a sweat, and couldn't believe that anyone could reverse the effects of aging to such an extent. As David parted ways with him at the 12-mile marker, the old guy was practically sprinting up the side trail to another lookout point. "If I don't see the view today, I'll just have to come back tomorrow," he called out. The lesson is simple: Exercise may or may not add more years to your life, but it certainly adds more life to your years.

- Sip water and nibble food frequently. Drink water every 15 minutes if your walk will be longer than an hour; snacks are a must for ventures of two hours or more.
- Set a moderate tempo, but keep moving consistently. Stop as often as you need for food and water, but don't dawdle. The tale of the hare and the tortoise was never truer than on the trail. A consistent, moderate pace will cover more ground than hasty bursts followed by long collapses to recover. It will be a lot more pleasant, too.
- Look up from the trail often. Don't just put your nose down and grind; lift your head a lot to see where you're going and

where you've been—you'll probably surprise yourself. Take a camera; enjoy the views.

- In a group, let the slowest walker set the pace. If that's just too slow for some of you, then break into smaller groups of similar ability and plan to join up at intervals—say, every 45 minutes—for a snack stop. Just don't let someone end up all alone behind the group—it can be no fun, and even dangerous.

- Set a turn-back time. Figure out half of the total time you're willing to be on the trail, and set that as the time you'll head back. Then here's the tough part: Stick with your time, even if you haven't reached your goal. The peak, waterfall, or view will be there for another hike—your job is to make sure that you are, too.

Make Every Walk Better: Warm-Ups and Cool-Downs

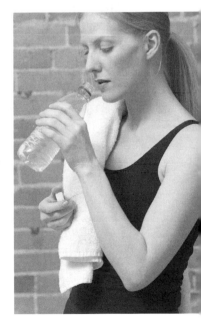

Warm-ups and cool-downs aren't just for big-time athletes. As you add steps to your day and distance to your walks, you'll find it helpful to include short warm-up and cool-down sessions, too. The prewalk moves below help you gradually increase the flow of blood to your muscles and joints, and reduce the risk of injury. Bottom line: You'll walk more comfortably and enjoy it more.

At the end of your walk, slow your pace for a few minutes. This gradual winding down helps avoid the cramping muscles and light-headed feeling that can come when your body doesn't gradually bring blood back to its core. Finish up with a few stretches while your muscles are warm and compliant to maintain flexibility and reduce the chance of injury. And talk about cheap—you get all this improved performance and reduced injury risk for a 10-minute total investment.

Five-Minute Warm-Up Routine

These should all be comfortable, unforced movements. Rest a hand on something for balance if necessary.

- **Ankle circles.** Stand on one foot and lift the other off the ground. Slowly flex that ankle through its full range of motion, making large circles with your toes, but only by moving your ankle joint, not your lower leg. Do six to eight in each direction, then switch feet and repeat.
- **Leg swings.** Stand on one leg, and swing the other loosely from your hip, front to back. It should be a relaxed, unforced motion like the swinging of a pendulum, and your foot should swing no higher than a foot or so off the ground. Do 15 to 20 swings on each leg.
- **Pelvic loops.** Put your hands on your hips with your knees "soft" (slightly bent) and feet shoulder width apart. Keep your body upright and make 10 slow continuous circles with your hips, pushing them gently forward, to the left, back, and to the right. Then reverse directions and repeat.
- **Arm circles.** Hold both arms straight out to the sides, making yourself into a letter *T*. Make 10 to 12 slow backward circles with your hands, starting small and finishing with large circles, using your entire arm. Shake your arms out,

then repeat with 10 to 12 slow forward circles, again starting small and getting larger.

- **Hula-hoop jumps.** Begin by jumping in place on both feet.
Keep your head and shoulders facing forward, and twist your
feet and lower body left then right, back and forth on succes-
sive jumps. Jump 15 to 20 times, facing forward but twisting
your hips and legs left and right on alternate jumps.

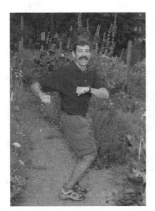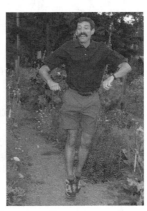

Mark Fenton thinks looking goofy is a small price to pay for
the great total body warm-up of Hula-hoop jumps.

- **Up, side, back, downs.** A great warm-up, but also ideal if
you ever experience shin soreness while walking. Stand
with your feet hip width apart and roll your feet through
four positions, holding each for a two-count. Start with six
repetitions, but build up to 10 to 15 sets.
Up. Stand on your toes, heels as high as possible.
Side. Roll to the outside edges of your feet, with the inside
edges pulled up.
Back. Stand on your heels, with your toes held as high as
possible.
Down. Rest, with both feet flat on the floor.

Five-Minute Postwalk Stretch Routine

You may have never had the flexibility of a prima ballerina, but it is still worth doing just a few minutes of stretching after each walk when your muscles are the most warm and elastic. That's enough to help maintain your mobility and a healthy range of movement for a lifetime of active living. It's also likely to reduce the chance of injuries. Here are four simple, stand-up stretches you can do anyplace, anytime after a walk.

Do all of these stretches slowly, never to the point of discomfort, and hold each stretch for six to eight slow, deep breaths. Imagine releasing muscle tension with each cleansing exhale. Begin each stretch standing up, and feel free to rest one hand on something for balance if necessary. If you have time, go through the cycle twice.

- **Calf and hip stretch.** Take a giant step forward with your left foot. Bend your left knee so your left shin is vertical (but don't push it beyond your foot) and keep your right heel on the ground and your right leg straight behind you. Stand tall, extending the crown of your head to the sky, and keep your abdominal muscles gently contracted so there's no excess arch in your back. You 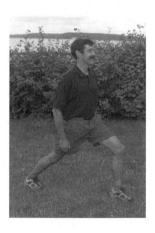 should feel the stretch in both your right calf *and* hip. Hold for several deep breaths. Then switch legs and repeat.
- **Back and hamstring stretch.** Take a small step forward with your left foot, straighten your left leg, and lift your toes upward. Keep your right foot flat on the ground, bend your

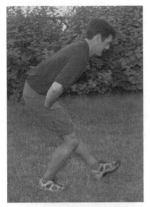

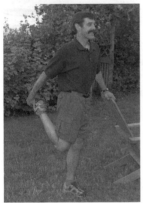

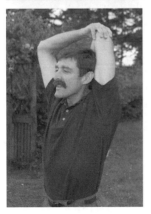

right knee slightly, set your hips back a bit, and hinge forward from your hips. Keep your back flat and chest forward, and feel the stretch in your back and the back of your left thigh. Look at your right toes, pulling them up for more stretch or easing them down for less. Hold for several deep breaths. Then switch legs and repeat.

- **Shin and thigh stretch.** Grasp your right toes with your right hand, and gently pull your foot up behind you, keeping your right knee pointed toward the ground. Your heel does not have to reach your buttocks—just pull to the point of feeling a gentle stretch in the front of the thigh, hip, and shin. Hold for several deep breaths. Then switch legs and repeat.

- **Shoulder and back.** Standing tall, point your left arm toward the ceiling, then bend your left elbow so your hand is behind your head. Grasp your left elbow with your right hand, and gently pull to the right. Hold for six slow breaths. Switch arms and repeat.

STEPS TO SUCCESS

Measuring Trail Miles

When you're hiking, a pedometer that displays both steps and distance can be helpful on trails where signposts are few and far between. Don't expect rock-solid accuracy—your stride length changes when you go up and down hills and deal with uneven footing. But on better trails with a mix of terrain, a pedometer can reliably estimate distances to within 5 to 10 percent of the posted trail values. Combined with good map and compass skills, those estimates from a pedometer can help you measure your progress and keep track of where you actually are.

How to Choose Hiking Boots

Unless you're planning a multiday adventure or you'll be carrying a heavy overnight pack, your best bet is a pair of so-called light hikers. They come in low-, mid-, and high-cut styles. Higher-cut styles offer more coverage and support, but tend to be a bit heavier and warmer than lower-cut models. Here's what to consider:

- **Fit.** This is your number one priority. What feels like a little slipping at the store can turn into a giant blister after an hour on the trail. The heel shouldn't slip when you step, and your toes should never touch the front of the shoe. If there's an incline in the store, walk up and down it, or jam your feet hard on a carpeted surface to make sure your toes won't get scrunched when you walk downhill. There should be no pinching or binding at the widest part of your foot, especially when you push off.
- **Protection underfoot.** Thick, lugged soles protect your feet from rocks and roots underfoot. Keep in mind that a beefier sole delivers more protection, but usually at the price of greater weight and stiffness.

STEPS TO SUCCESS

10 Essentials for Your Day Pack

Whether you plan to spend a couple of hours on a nearby wooded nature trail or devote a day to tackling a summit, play it safe by stowing these items in your pack. If hiking gets to be a habit, just have numbers 3 through 10 in your pack always ready to go.

1. Water. Enough for the hike, plus an extra bottle.
2. Food. Lunch, plus some high-energy food (peanuts, a sports bar, chocolate).
3. Weather gear. In summer, pack a hat, sunscreen, and insect repellent. In spring or fall or if you're bound for higher altitudes, bring a rain jacket and extra layers.
4. First-aid kit. A minimum supply includes aspirin and acetaminophen, several sizes of adhesive bandages and gauze pads, disinfectant, Ace bandages, athletic tape, and safety pins.
5. Trail map and compass. If you'll be walking for more than a couple of miles or leaving signed trails, be sure you know how to use them.
6. Whistle. Three loud blasts followed by a pause is the universal signal for help.
7. Water purification tablets (generally iodine).
8. Simple pocketknife. Ideally one with an opener, screwdriver, tweezers, and scissors.
9. Lighter (or at least dry matches) and a candle stub for starting an emergency fire.
10. Small flashlight or headlamp and extra batteries. If you fall behind schedule, this can be the thing that gets you back to the car without a twisted ankle.

- **Ankle support.** If you have weak ankles, are negotiating tricky terrain, or are wearing a heavy pack (say, carrying all the lunches, emergency gear, and more), a higher-cut ankle boot is a good choice. Low- and midcut models are designed for smooth trails and more moderate terrain.

- **Waterproofing.** Gore-Tex and other waterproof materials are worth the investment for consistently cold, wet conditions. But for dew-covered fields and the occasional stream splash or light rain, you can do without, and your feet will be much cooler for it.
- **Traction.** Both the softness of the rubber and the depth of the treads come into play here. Softer materials offer great grip on slick rocks and the like, but wear out faster. Deeper treads hold well on rough terrain, dirt, and gravel, but add weight and stiffness. So go with a deeper tread on rougher trails, but less tread on more groomed pathways.

STEP BOOSTER

For every hour that you're relaxing at the beach, walk or swim for at least 20 minutes.

Expect a pair of hiking boots to give 400 to 600 miles of service, depending on the ruggedness of the trails you walk. One sure way to extend the life of walking or hiking shoes: Dry them thoroughly if they become very wet. But don't use heat to dry footwear, because it can damage the glues that are used. Instead, pull out the inner sole (if it's removable) and stuff the shoe with newspaper overnight to absorb the moisture.

Week Four Program

It's possible that you've found all the incidental steps you need to get your 10,000 steps a day. You know every stairwell at work, and have a reputation for striding across parking lots all over the county. But if a 10,000-step total (or higher, if you're looking for faster weight loss) is elusive, it may be time to actually thrust a structured walk or other exercise into your day. We've suggested several ways to make it happen—hooking up with others through a walking group, training for a weekend walking event, or weaving a hike somewhere into your week.

But you can sure make it simpler if you want to. If heading out the door for a quick 20-minute jaunt first thing in the morning does the trick for you, then stride on. Or if an after-dinner walking meditation makes life calm and balanced, then get out and commune with the stars. We just offered these more structured avenues to more steps for those who are finding stepping it up

STEP BOOSTER

Try orienteering, a sport requiring use of a map and compass to navigate through designated checkpoints in the woods. (Even kids love it.)

either challenging, or simply not that much fun. Walking with others, participating in an event, or taking a hike will definitely boost your step total, and most people find at least one of those ideas pretty enjoyable.

So if you can manage it, give at least one a try this week. Nothing earth shattering—just hook up with a lunchtime walking group at work or sign up for the fund-raising walk in your city this weekend. If you keep doing everything else that's already working, you may find that one of these things, combined with, say, a Wednesday-afternoon hike in a nearby park, is all you need to get your 20 percent boost for the week. And remember, even as you measure your daily step totals to chart your progress and stay motivated, try to also be aware of your weekly total. That allows for the occasional low-step day by letting you get back on track with a few step-heavier days to still hit your goal for the week.

Week Four Step Log

Number of steps	Anything special today?
Monday	
Tuesday	
Wednesday	
Thursday	
Friday	
Saturday	
Sunday	
Week Total	

Daily average: _____
(total steps for the week divided by 7)

Daily goal for next week: _____
(daily average x 1.2, for a 20% increase)

Week Five

More Steps, Less Time

The closer you get to your step goal, the harder you're likely to find it is to add more steps. After all, if you started at a fairly typical level—say, 5,000 steps a day—then the first week you were only trying to add 1,000 steps, or about 10 minutes of walking a day. But if you've added anything near to 20 percent a week, you're closing in on a daily goal of 10,000 steps or more. And frankly, it's pretty normal to find it hard to *keep* adding steps—after all, that's almost an additional hour of activity over your original 5,000 steps, even if it is spread throughout the day. Fortunately, the answer may be easier than you think: Start making just some of those steps faster, and you'll not only squeeze them into less time, but also boost the calorie-burning and fitness-building benefits.

STEPS TO SUCCESS

**Racewalking—
The Speediest Way to More Steps**

If you've ever seen real, elite competitive racewalkers—not just the Chaplin-esque caricatures—then you know the motion is actually very smooth, efficient, and athletic. To be competitive, it has to be. Top competitors can cover 20 kilometers in less than an hour and a half. That's 12.4 miles at a speedy pace of 7 minutes, 20 seconds per mile—better than 8 miles an hour, and a tempo most runners would be delighted to match. The competitors in a 50-kilometer event (31 miles) *walk* a marathon in less than 3 hours, 30 minutes, and then hold that pace for another 5 miles.

The rules are actually pretty straightforward: A racewalker must maintain unbroken contact with the ground (the obvious difference between a walk and a run), and the knee of the supporting leg must be straight at heel contact (this assures none of the benefits of a "springy" knee that makes running so much faster than walking). Judges circle the course and remove competitors after three infractions of those rules.

Not surprisingly, when top racewalkers were tested at the U.S. Olympic Training Center in Colorado Springs, they were seen to have fitness levels comparable to those of elite runners. Body fat, endurance, maximal oxygen uptake, and lactate thresholds (if you're into that sort of thing) were similar for the runners and racewalkers. Yet racewalkers appear to suffer fewer of the impact-related injuries experienced by many runners, as walkers only strike the ground with 1.0 to 1.5 times their body weight, while runners slam to earth with 3.0 or more times their body weight on every stride.

The final bonus? Typical racewalking speeds garner step rates of 160 steps per minute or more; elites are clocked at roughly 200 steps a minute. Learn to racewalk at high speed, and you could muster 1,000 steps in just five minutes at a blazing pace. Even better, get a full day's 10,000-step allotment in less than an hour!

(See "Racewalking" in the Resources section for more information.)

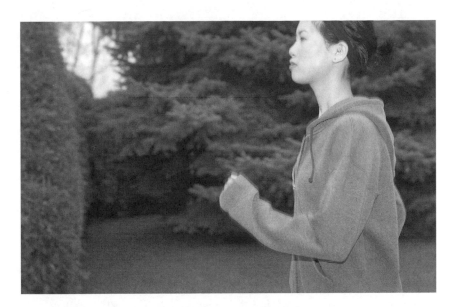

Quick Steps to the Rescue

Picking up the pace is a great way to get more steps done in less time. Whether you're going out for an actual workout, or just walking from the subway to work, it follows that you'll get more steps in fewer minutes if you're walking faster.

Is there any other upside to faster walking? Well, everything you get *some* of from walking at slower speeds, you get *lots* of from faster walking. Walk at a comfortable, chatting pace and burn maybe 250 Calories an hour. Crank it up to a brisk walk and burn 350 to 400 Calories in the same amount of time. Walk slowly and reduce your risk for chronic illnesses such as cardiovascular disease and diabetes. But regularly make your walks vigorous, and see a dramatic rise in the likelihood of a longer, healthier life. And to improve your cardiorespiratory fitness—that ability to dash up a flight of stairs or play sports without buckling over, hands on knees, gasping for air—research suggests you need three or more outings of vigorous walking a week. These faster walks strengthen your heart and fortify your muscles, building greater blood vessel density and helping to create more energy production sites (called mitochondria) at the cellular level. Pretty good payoff for simply walking fast enough to get yourself breathing hard a few times a week, don't you think?

The problem is that many people simply feel they can't walk fast enough to boost their heart rate or actually get themselves breathing noticeably. It's the *walking-can't-really-be-a-workout* syndrome. Fortunately, we have four simple tips that will have anyone walking at a fitness-building pace in no time at all. They're gleaned from the technical form of competitive racewalkers, but simplified so that they're easy to master and, frankly, look nothing

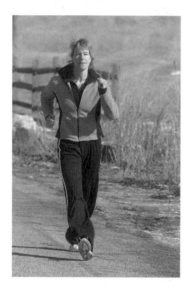

like the exaggerated arm action or hip sway that dissuades many would-be fitness walkers.

Four Tips for Faster Walking

To boost your walking to a speed that's sure to build fitness and burn calories, and garner lots of steps, you don't have to be a racewalker. Just learn from them. Try these four simple tips to pick your walk up to a more aerobic pace.

1. **Stand tall.** No slouch in your shoulders, forward lean from the waist, or excess sway in your lower back. Keep your

chin level, and feel as if a string is extending from your spine and pulling you upward through the top of your head.

Cue: Keep your eyes on the horizon. Lower your eyes to check your footing, of course, but don't drop your chin.

2. **Focus on quicker, not longer steps.** Sure, your stride gets longer as you walk faster. But that shouldn't be your goal; let it happen naturally. Concentrate instead on taking *faster* steps. Try counting your steps for just 20 seconds, working to hit the rough benchmarks of 40 (health), 45 (weight loss) or 50 (fitness) steps. They're equal to 120, 135, and 150 steps per minute, respectively.

   Cue: Try this experiment. Stand tall with your feet together. Then shift your weight to the balls of your feet and slowly lean forward from the ankles. Keep your body straight until you naturally feel the need to step forward to catch yourself. The step you take is a good indication of your starting stride length for a moderate speed.

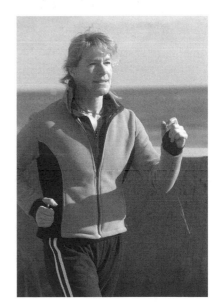

3. **Bend your arms.** Hold your elbows at a right angle so your arms can swing more quickly. A short pendulum swings more easily than a long one, so target a quick, compact arm swing.

PEDOMETER PRO
Presidential Pedometry

Harry S. Truman, U.S. president from 1945 to 1953, was an avid early-morning walker. With his trademark hat and cane, he would set off along the streets of Washington, DC, with reporters and Secret Service men scrambling to keep up. A Washington admirer sent Truman a pedometer engraved with the words, FOR PRESIDENT TRUMAN AND HIS STEPS FORWARD. Truman replied in a letter, "The very next morning after I received it I rung up two and one-half miles on it. I appreciate your sending it to me because now I can keep track of just how far I go."

After his presidency Truman returned home to Missouri, where he continued his walking. He published his memoirs and remained active in politics until his death at 88 years of age. When asked for his advice for a long life, Truman replied, "Take a brisk 2-mile walk before breakfast every morning." Never one for a leisurely stroll, "Give-em-Hell Harry" further recommended, "You should always walk as though you have someplace to go." Good advice for anyone looking to boost step totals, and to all hoping to live a long and vigorous life.

(Think about it this way—how many runners do you see out there running with straight arms?) Don't let your elbows flail out to the sides, or have your hands come up to chin (or even nose) height in front.

Cue: Your hands should trace an arc from alongside your waistband on the backswing, to chest height (no higher) in the front.

4. Push off with your toes. Consciously extend your ankle fully on each step, pushing off with your toes aggressively and generating as much boost as possible at the end of each stride.

Cue: You should roll the foot all the way through your toes, and feel like you're showing someone behind you the bottom of your shoe on every step.

The Real Skinny on Burning Calories

Lots of exercise machines at the gym (such as treadmills and rowing machines) and more and more pedometers purport to tell you how many calories you're burning while exercising. It's fine to take note of these as encouragement for your good effort, but be sure to take the absolute figures with a big grain of salt. That's because there are a tremendous number of factors that really influence how many calories you burn during exercise. An indoor machine should at least account for your age, gender, body weight, fitness level, and effort (best measured by your heart rate) to have a shot at estimating your caloric expenditure. Take the exercise outside and you can add terrain and weather conditions to the confounding factors. That's why pedometers can really only offer rough estimates for calories burned—especially if they don't account for at least your weight and effort level (by measuring both your steps and how fast you're taking them).

However, you can get a calorie burn estimate that's at least that accurate simply with a step-counting pedometer and your watch. All you have to do is calculate your steps per minute for a walk (the total number of steps you took divided by the time you walked, in minutes) and know your body weight:

$$\text{Step Rate (in steps per minute)} = \frac{\text{Total Steps Taken}}{\text{Time for the Walk (in minutes)}}$$

Then the two tables on pages 90 and 91 will quickly get you to an estimate of the calories you expended during a walk. Of course, don't go using a good 500-Calorie walk as justification for eating a hot fudge sundae the size of your head, but rather as motivation to get in another great walk tomorrow.

Accurately Estimating Your Walking Speed

It's possible to estimate your speed based on your rate of steps per minute. Divide the total number of steps you take during a specific walk by the total number of minutes the walk took. Then go down the column for your height range, and find the estimate of your average speed for the walk. So, if Bob is 6 feet, 2 inches tall, and took 3,452 steps in a 25-minute walk, he calculates:

$$\frac{3,452}{25} = 138$$

He averaged about 138 steps per minute. Looking down the table under "greater than 6 feet," he sees that falls between 130 and 140 steps per minute, or a swift 4.5 miles per hour.

Step Rate and Estimated Walking Speeds

Step Rate (Steps/Minute)			Time to Walk 1 Mile (Min:Sec)	Estimated Walking Speed (mph)
If You're < 5'6"	If You're 5'6" to 6'	If You're > 6'		
100–110	95–105	90–100	30:00	2.0
105–115	100–110	95–105	24:00	2.5
110–120	105–115	100–110	20:00	3.0
120–130	115–125	110–120	17:10	3.5
130–140	125–135	120–130	15:00	4.0
140–150	135–145	130–140	13:20	4.5
155–165	150–160	145–155	12:00	5.0

These rough speed estimates are great to use in estimating the calories you've burned, with the next table (below).

Getting from Speed to Calorie Burn

With the walking speed you've gotten based on your step rate, you can use this table to estimate the calories you burn while walking for 30 minutes; use the weight column that's closest to yours, or estimate between the two closest values. This is for level ground in normal weather conditions; a hilly walk or very windy day could boost your effort sub-

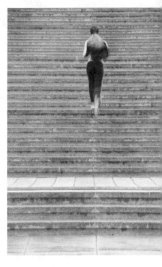

stantially. Cruising up just a modest incline of 6 percent (that's climbing just 6 feet for every 100 feet that you walk forward) will boost the caloric expenditure by 16 percent; crank up to a very noticeable incline (say, 10 percent, or 1 foot of climb for every 10 feet forward) and calories burned grows by more than 50 percent, even if you slow down a bit.

Estimated Calorie Burn for 30 Minutes of Walking

Speed (mph)	Body Weight					
	100 lbs.	125 lbs.	150 lbs.	175 lbs.	200 lbs.	250 lbs.
2.0	63	80	95	110	126	158
2.5	73	92	110	128	147	183
3.0	86	108	129	151	172	215
3.5	103	128	154	180	205	257
4.0	125	156	187	218	250	311
4.5	154	193	231	270	308	385
5.0	196	245	293	342	391	490

STEPPING STONE

Quick Calories Per Mile

If this seems too complicated, remember this quick-and-easy rule of thumb: To estimate how many calories you'll burn per mile walked, simply divide your body weight in pounds by 2. Example: You weigh 140 pounds. So, 140 / 2 = 70 Calories burned per mile. This works pretty well for walking speeds ranging from 2 to 4 mph.

Calorie estimates arrived at by different means really can't be compared. Don't expect the treadmill at a gym and this table to give you the same calorie estimates, even for identical-length walks of similar effort. But if you use a standard method—say, a pedometer or heart rate monitor—you can at least compare the estimate from one workout to the next to see how you're doing.

Steer Clear of Hand Weights, Vests, and Stretch Cords

Hand weights are often marketed as an easy way to add an upper-body punch to the cardiovascular workout of walking, but as a general rule we don't recommend using them. To get the best workout with hand weights, you have to bend your elbows and pump your arms vigorously, and if you maintain your walking speed while carrying hand weights you might increase the calories you burn by anywhere from 10 to 50 percent. But research suggests that a 5 to 20 percent increase is more likely if you're carrying a reasonable amount of weight (less than 10 percent of your body weight). Keep in mind that this assumes you're not slowing down, which can happen quite easily with the weights in your hands. And you can get at least half of that increase in energy expenditure simply by bending your arms 90 degrees and pumping them vigorously—without weights—during a brisk walk.

Hand weights can also bring concerns for people who have a history of shoulder or elbow problems or postural issues, or for anyone with heart trouble or high blood pressure. The latter is because the act of gripping the weights can boost your blood pressure somewhat artificially, an effect called the pressor response.

Another intensity booster on the market is a weighted vest. The idea is that adding weights to pockets on the vest will make you work harder and burn off more fat. The problem is that carrying weight close to your torso is really quite efficient—it's why soldiers and backpackers learn to load their backpacks with the heaviest materials close to their bodies, where they induce the least extra effort. Though a weighted vest can really bump up the burn in aerobics and step classes where you tend to move up and down a lot, given the amount of weight you'd have to pile on to make a difference, it's probably not worth the aggravation when out walking.

> **STEP BOOSTER**
>
> Play hopscotch. Keep trying until you don't miss.

A third device designed to intensify walking is a hip belt with retractable cords that you pull while vigorously swinging your arms. Developed by cross-country skiers, and used in aerobics classes and the like to challenge the upper body, these belts are not necessarily easy to master when walking. They require a good deal of coordination, and can be plenty awkward at first. But lest you think we're purist snobs, and down on all possible adjuncts to walking, you'll find that we think one in particular is worth considering.

Boost Your Workout with Nordic Walking

You may have noticed in the "How Active Are America's Favorite Activities?" table in Week Four that cross-country (or Nordic) skiing had the highest typical calorie burn for 30 minutes. That's no coincidence. Nordic skiing is a low-impact activity that utilizes all the major muscle groups of the body in large repetitive movements that are challenging, but not damaging. Once you get fit, you can do it for literally hours and not suffer injury.

It should be no surprise, then, that for years Nordic skiers have been using their ski poles while walking and running—even when

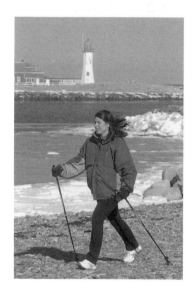

there's no snow on the ground—to stay in shape for ski season. Hikers, too, are accustomed to using one or two poles when crossing rugged terrain to help maintain balance, especially when carrying full loads. Hiking poles also help ease the pounding on knees and ankles when you're hiking downhill.

So it was only a matter of time before someone decided to turn this into a formal exercise. Termed Nordic walking by its promoters, the idea is simply to walk while using superlight poles in a cross-country skiing motion with your arms. You step with your right foot while poling with your left arm, and vice versa. Before you chuckle, hear the upside: Studies show that Nordic walking can burn from 15 to 45 percent more calories than normal walking, and it does effectively engage the muscles of the chest, back, shoulders, arms, and abdomen. Once you master poling vigorously, it can be especially good for the lats (latissimus dorsi, the "wing" muscles under the arms) and triceps, or back of the upper arm (a problem spot for many women).

Originally, only heavier, adjustable-length poles designed for hiking were available for Nordic walking. However, with its rise

PEDOMETER PRO

Applause for Paws

An Australian study showed that dog owners who walked their dogs took about 2,000 steps more than those who did not—10,900 versus 9,000 steps per day. And when you consider how busy some dogs are, you can see how helping your Rover get enough exercise can quickly benefit you, too.

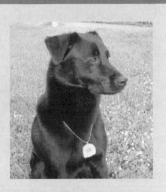

To examine this more closely, we found a special pedometer that's made in Japan just for dogs. Turns out coauthor David Bassett's three-year-old Lab-chow, Tubby, averages 38,000 steps per day, and would probably take more if he could. (Talk about picking up the pace!) Tubby's favorite ways to get more steps? Carousing with his canine buddies at the nearby park, playing Frisbee, and taking 3-mile walks around the neighborhood with any willing member of his family. Which begs the question: Why in the world is this dog called Tubby?

in popularity, manufacturers are now making lightweight, superstrong Nordic walking poles. They're fixed length with a graphite-composite shaft, Nordic-ski-type handgrips and wrist straps for comfort, and removable rubber tips for use on paved surfaces. (They're removed to reveal a metal spike tip for use on grass, sand, dirt trails, and other softer surfaces.)

Notably, we've found that when we Nordic walk, we actually tend to walk faster. Even though a lot more calories are burned, research shows that the rate of perceived exertion (that's physiologist talk for "how hard it feels") doesn't go up commensurately. They suspect that's because the workload is spread over more of

STEPS TO SUCCESS

Rover to the Rescue

If you're having trouble getting out the door to exercise, you just might be in need of a canine personal trainer. Dr. Robert Kushner, professor of medicine at Northwestern University in Chicago, led a study of overweight pets and their owners. He enrolled 56 people, some with dogs, in a diet and exercise program. The people were encouraged to walk at least 20 minutes per day and restrict themselves to 1,400 Calories per day. (The dogs were fed a special prescription diet made by 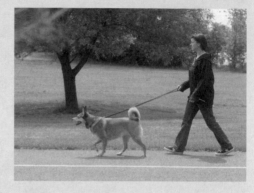 Hill's Pet Nutrition, which funded the study.) After a year, the people and dogs had both lost an average of about 11 pounds. When people and their pets exercised together, they had more success. Sometimes a dog really is its owner's best friend!

your body—not just legs, but arms and torso muscles, too. So it's likely that the poling action is actually helping to propel you along—certainly making for a harder effort, but one that you're able to handle. And how does that work from a pedometric standpoint? Well, anything that helps you get in more steps in less time is a good thing, if you ask us.

Week Five Program

Okay, the equation is simple: The faster you walk, the more steps you get and the less time it takes. Plus, with several faster walks a week you get boosted fitness benefits, and you burn more calories in less time. So this week the goal is not to add a lot more walking time to your days. It's to add a lot more steps to your walking time. Here's how it works.

First, for all the incidental steps you add to your week—climbing stairs instead of taking the elevator, doing errands on foot—try to move at a comfortably brisk pace. Obviously, if you're carrying groceries or walking to work, you may not be able or want to go at a full-fledged arm-swinging, sweat-inducing aerobic pace. But no dawdling. Moving briskly will assure that these incidental steps, while adding to your daily total, won't take quite as much time.

Second, for the times that you consciously go out specifically just to walk, try to really pick up the pace at least three times this week. You don't have to kill yourself, but use all four elements of speedy walking technique: tall posture, quick steps, bent arms, and pushing off with your toes. Try this for at least 10 minutes, or about 1,300 to 1,500 steps' worth of speedier walking each time. If improved aerobic fitness—and the weight loss and health benefits that come with it—is one of your goals, then you should eventually work up to a brisk 20-minute walk, or 2,600 to 3,000 steps' worth, three days a week. And whatever else you do, keep working toward at least an average of 10,000 steps per day, or 70,000 steps per week.

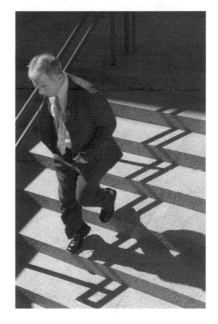

Week Five Step Log

Number of steps	Anything special today?
Monday	
Tuesday	
Wednesday	
Thursday	
Friday	
Saturday	
Sunday	
Week Total	

Daily average: _____
(total steps for the week divided by 7)

Daily goal for next week: _____
(daily average x 1.2, for a 20% increase)

Week Six

Get Serious

Your pedometer is no longer a novelty item, and frankly, you may think you have this thing figured out by now. Here's the problem—five weeks of success does not an active lifetime make. To put it more bluntly, the question isn't whether you can boost your daily steps for five weeks or even five months. The question is whether you can do it for the next five years, then 15, and then hopefully 50 more after that. It's not about whether you can build up to 10,000 or 12,000 steps a day, it's about whether you can stay there.

Unfortunately—and you probably won't be surprised to learn this—health professionals regularly quote a statistic that more

STEPPING STONE

Are We *Really* Becoming Less Active?

Most Americans feel that it's harder than ever to keep the weight off, and many researchers believe that our modern, busy lifestyles are to blame. We reviewed data from a variety of sources, and it does indeed seem that Americans have become less active since 1960. National time-use surveys show a decline in time spent preparing meals (44 minutes then versus 27 now) and meal cleanup (21 versus 4). And Department of Labor statistics show that fewer people today have strenuous jobs such as farming and manual labor compared with 40 years ago.

We all see evidence of myriad ways to burn just a few less calories everywhere around us, from remote-control garage door openers and televisions, to leaf blowers and sit-down lawn mowers; from dishwashers and microwaves to escalators and suitcases on wheels. And Americans now spend a lot more of their free time watching TV, surfing the Internet, or playing video games. A recent cartoon by Skelton shows a dad lecturing his teenage son, who's sitting on the couch with the TV remote control. "Why, when I was your age I had to walk 10 feet to change the channels!" exclaims the dad. This decline in lifestyle physical activity has been partly offset by increased participation in exercise routines (especially in women), but the blossoming obesity epidemic suggests that this offset is not nearly enough.

The International Obesity Task Force, not one for mincing words, sums up this losing battle very simply as the result of a two-pronged attack: an environment that limits our chances to be physically active, and an oversupply of calorie-dense foods and drinks, leading to chronic overconsumption. Sounds like another 2,000 steps are in order, doesn't it?

than half of the people who start a new fitness program drop out within the first six months, and three-quarters drop out within the first year. So, will you be a dropout, or will you find a way to make more steps permanently and inalienably part of your life going forward? First, you should seriously consider wearing your pedometer beyond this six-week program—many people find it a critical motivator and tool for long-term success. But to really make it stick, you may have to think about more than your own habits. You may have to think about your whole community.

The French Vacation Paradox

We're amazed at how often we hear this story: A friend comes back from a two-week vacation in Europe—say, Paris—and raves about the great trip and amazing food. She goes on to describe how she ate whatever she wanted whenever she wanted, and never passed up dessert. And yet she's stunned—shocked—to have actually lost two, or four, or we've even heard *seven* pounds while over there. It's a paradox—how can it be?

So we ask—where did you stay? "Right in the city, of course." And what did you do? "Saw every museum, historical site, great cathedral . . . We did it all." And what kind of car did you rent? "Oh, we didn't rent a car. We walked everywhere; took the subway or train for longer trips . . ." You get the picture.

Undoubtedly less between-meal snacking, saner portion sizes, and longer days may have contributed to the weight loss. But given the typical vacation diet, it's fairly certain that the increased activity level was critical to the change. It's also a key reason why French women purportedly don't get fat (and might explain why the recent book of the same title is a best seller). Here's the big "secret"—our friend probably walked 15,000 to 20,000 steps a day on that vacation, easily two to five times the activity she got back home in the United States. In fact, research suggests Europeans walk about 250 miles per person per year (this is just what researchers call *functional* walking to destinations, rather than fitness walking) compared with 90 miles per person per year in the

U.S. In the Netherlands and Denmark, people bicycle an additional 550 miles per person per year! This compares with only 25 miles of average bicycling in America.

All of this adds up to Europeans burning 60 to 120 Calories per person per day through physically active transportation, compared with only 20 Calories in the U.S. It's reasonable to suspect this is an important contributing factor in explaining why obesity rates are much higher in the United States than Europe.

Unfortunately, even though this empirical data may help explain why French women don't get fat, it doesn't seem to be enough. As American lifestyles are increasingly adopted in Europe and the rest of the world—from the rise of fast food to more households having two cars and driving to more destinations—obesity rates are climbing across the globe. And a decline in active commuting—walking or biking to work or the train—is likely a contributing factor.

Walking as a Way of Life

Here's a list of ways we could build more steps into everyday life in America. Though some seem outlandish now, none of them would have seemed at all extreme just 50 years ago.

- Walk your kids to and from school every day.
- Take mass transit—a bus, train, or trolley—to work, and walk or bike to and from the station at both ends of the trip.
- Walk to the corner store for milk and bread.
- Pick up your mail at a post office box.
- Have only one car in your household, and—true blasphemy—a one-car garage.

- Live close enough to a bank, school, post office, shopping, and work that it seems reasonable to your parents and children to actually do all of this walking.
- Have only one television in your house.
- Don't subscribe to cable televison (and scores, perhaps hundreds, of viewing options at all times).
- Don't drive the kids everywhere they need to go. Most of all, don't drive them to the mall.

The question is, can we really create environments in this day and age that don't make the list above look like an idyllic fantasy? Without a doubt, we can. Communities across America from big cities to tiny villages and even rural areas—many under threat of being overrun by development—are making decisions every day to build places where it's easy, and even desirable to get out and walk regularly. The efforts fall into four major categories; they're based

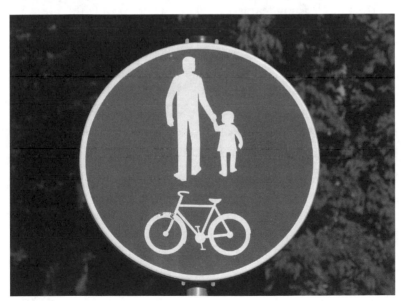

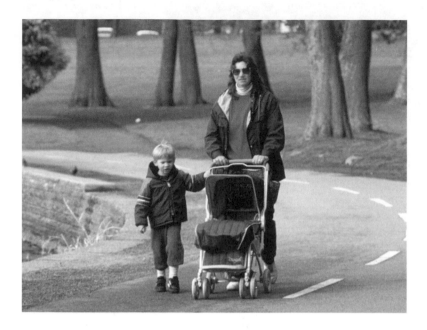

on the four defining features of places where people tend to walk and bicycle more and drive less.

1. *Mixed-Use and Compact Zoning*

Many communities are changing their planning and land-use codes to encourage neighborhoods that look less like cookie-cutter subdivisions and strip malls, and more like traditional neighborhoods. Many codes encouraged sprawl through "single-use" zoning, requiring housing, retail, and commercial areas to be separate. The result was housing over here, shopping malls there, office parks and a school out there, and a ride in the car to get from any one to another.

But new alternatives have tremendous appeal: Downtowns have retail stores on the first floor and offices and apartments above. Residential areas have corner stores and civic buildings—

libraries, schools, and post offices—right in the mix. And lot sizes tend to be smaller, which shortens the walking distance between destinations. The benefit is that rather than each home having a giant underused yard, open space is collected in more beneficial greenbelts and trails, parks and playing fields.

2. Complete Pedestrian and Bicycle Networks

This ranges from the mundane—sidewalks and safe street crossings—to the magnificent, such as waterfront trails, boardwalks, and bikeways.

Sidewalks, and not just cruddy ones, on every street are a must. They should be five or more feet wide and separated from roadways, with a planting strip and ideally even what experts call "street furniture," which includes everything from trees to benches. Further, many roads need painted bicycle lanes (they can improve driver and bicyclist behavior), and critical connections can be made with pathways and trails. A popular and highly successful approach is converting unused rail corridors into multiuse paths— called rails-to-trails—or placing trails alongside but safely segregated from active rail lines (rails-*with*-trails).

> **STEP BOOSTER**
>
> Trade in your riding lawn mower for a power push mower.

3. Step-Friendly Architecture

Building planners should stop designing buildings with stairways that are locked and alarmed so you can't just walk up one flight. They should go a step farther and mimic the Centers for Disease Control, which cleaned and carpeted the stairwells, put up art, and piped in music in the building housing their chronic disease prevention branch (where else?). The result was, not surprisingly, more folks climbing the stairs.

But the biggest item on our wish list is to make sure buildings welcome cyclists and pedestrians. Buildings should be up close to the street, not behind huge parking lots (put the parking out back or underneath). Entries should connect to sidewalks, and bicycle parking should be obvious, covered, plentiful, and secure. Homes should be nearer the street as well, with front porches the most prominent feature, and garages out back or on the side. The result is a street that feels and *is* safer and more inviting for walking.

4. Safety, Safety, Safety

Destinations can be close, connected by sidewalks, and architecture can be inviting, but if cars are blasting down the street at 45 miles an hour, people still won't walk and bike. Fortunately, engineers have a full tool kit of methods to "calm" traffic, slow speeds, and make crossing the street not an adventure, but a simple task. And it's not all about speed bumps. Clever devices such as median islands, curb extensions (or sidewalk "bump-outs"), special crosswalk markings and lights (even flashing lights in the pavement), narrowed lanes, and mini traffic circles in neighborhoods all help slow traffic and dramatically lessen the risks to pedestrians and drivers alike. Two more great perks of pedestrian-friendly street design: Crashes are reduced, and traffic tends to flow more smoothly.

> **STEP BOOSTER**
>
> Put up some bird feeders or birdhouses and keep them well stocked.

But what about someone who's chosen a more rural lifestyle? Sadly, evidence shows that it's a vanishing reality, with ever-increasing portions of the U.S. population ending up in suburbs or their offspring—exurbs. Many of these step-unfriendly places are just the next ring of mall and sprawl development even farther from city and town centers, and requiring even longer car rides to shop and work.

• • •

What good are ideas about land use and sidewalks? As you think about living a more active lifestyle, you will no doubt come to lifetime crossroads: switching jobs, choosing your children's school, or buying a new home, for example. It's worth factoring the four attributes above—nearby destinations, the presence of a network for walking, buildings and facilities that make walking easy, and safe roadways—into your decision. After all, if you're looking at two homes, but one would let you walk your child to school and the other would put you in the car every morning, isn't the step-friendly house the better choice? Of course, it's likely to be a bit more expensive, too—the National Association of Realtors reports that homes in more walkable settings are found to be more desirable to buyers. But that means it will hold its value better—and you'll be healthy and live long enough to enjoy that increased value, to boot!

Time for Extreme Measures

Let's say it's three months down the road, and you're still diligently wearing your step counter. You've done everything we've recommended, adding steps whenever possible, but you're still stuck at 9,436 steps a day, even though your goal was to get closer to 12,000. Even worse, the weight has stopped coming off and you feel you've hit a fitness plateau.

Maybe it's time to stop nibbling around the edges, and do something that will really make a difference. And before you read this list and

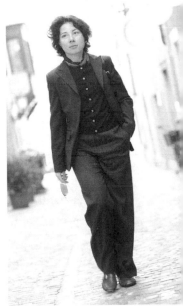

PEDOMETER PRO

Fred Kasch: The Payoff

Fred Kasch from San Diego, California, may not have relied on a pedometer to keep fit, but at age 92, he's living proof that staying active is a surefire way to enhance your quality of life as you age. A retired professor of physical education at San Diego State University, Kasch ran an adult fitness testing program through which he followed some members for more than 30 years. His data, which became landmark research, showed that men who remained active had lower blood pressures, resting heart rates, and body-fat levels, and also slowed the decline in aerobic fitness that comes with age.

An example of this himself, Kasch is still downhill skiing and deer hunting and alternates walking and jogging for 2 to 3 miles on most days, in addition to doing vigorous calisthenics. When he recently tracked his activity levels with a pedometer for 63 days, his records showed a daily average of nearly 4,500 steps a day, which did not include frequent dancing, hiking, wood chopping, and cycling. His additional notations—walk 0.75 miles to restaurant; saw wood, 30 minutes; walk to friend's house, 1.5 miles; run/walk 2.9 miles—indicate the kind of active life that make growing older something to look forward to.

say, *Well, who would do this stuff just to get more steps?* ask yourself these questions: How many people would move to a new city for a better-paying job? How many families would move to a different neighborhood for better schools? More to the point, how many people pay higher insurance premiums or even take a new job for better health coverage? If you think about the things we'd do for our own or our family's welfare, why shouldn't creating or moving to a more walkable community make the list?

With that appeal, here are some real things you can do to put more steps in your life and create a more step-friendly, healthy, livable community.

Walk with Seniors

Contact a local senior center and volunteer to walk with visitors or residents. It's possible to even offer to help seniors do errands on foot. Most important, of course, is the opportunity to simply visit and make some intergenerational contact—something sorely missing in much of our society.

Put on a Walking Event

Walking events are blossoming in popularity—even running-race directors admit that walkers make up an ever-growing portion of their participants. So why not organize a 2-mile fund-raiser for your church or school, or an afternoon educational walk with the historical society? Make it a regular monthly or weekly gig, and really lock in some steps.

Build a Trail

The good news is, you don't have to do it with your bare hands— although that can be the most fun. But trail building could range from helping to build or maintain a section of rugged, backcountry hiking path to working to get a section of old railroad right-of-way turned into a multiuse trail through a city or town (see "Walkable Communities" under Resources). Think about organizing locally—getting neighbors and friends interested in trails in and around your community. This boosts your effectiveness when you approach elected officials for support, property easements, and funding.

Make Your Workplace into a Walk Place

Recently companies have realized that increasing employee physical activity can reduce absenteeism and health costs, while improving

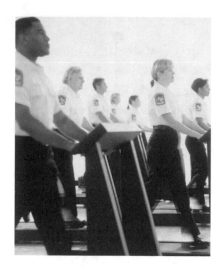

productivity and employee satisfaction. So help your boss make the connection between encouraging people to take more steps and the company's bottom line. Specific initiatives you can propose:

- Provide safe, covered bicycle parking, locker rooms, and showers for active commuters and lunch-hour workouts.
- Offer flex time; it eases the ability to take time out for a walk during the day, share in walk-to-school duties with kids, or build in time for commuting by bike or on foot.
- Open and clean stairwells; in bigger buildings, define hallway loops where folks can walk circuits indoors (during extreme weather); create trails or mark mileage and steps on outdoor pathways.

 STEPS TO SUCCESS

More Walking While You Work?

Maybe you've heard of the standing desks that are promoted to improve posture and back health. Well, how about putting a treadmill in front of one and accumulating steps while you compose e-mails and talk on the phone? Before you scoff, know that Dr. James Levine at the Mayo Clinic in Rochester, Minnesota, a researcher who's explored the impact of "burning calories by fidgeting," walks at 0.7 mph on the treadmill while working at his desk. It seems he's built the ultimately step-friendly office environment.

- Launch an employee walking program. Underwrite the cost of pedometers, create departmental teams, and give prizes.
- Get really wild, as the most innovative employers do, by subsidizing active commuting. Give away transit passes, pay people to walk and bike, but charge money for employee parking. Talk about a real step booster!

Wean Your Kids, Friends, and Colleagues Off the Chauffeur Service

Declare a moratorium on car rides to the school, mall, video store, or anywhere else that could be safely walked, biked, or bused, or skipped all together. For kids, this is a huge opportunity to reduce car time and increase active travel—after all, you can still walk or bike your child to a friend's or to soccer practice. But even adults are addicted to the car—think of the coworker who says, "Come on, I'll drive over to the other building for the meeting"—when often a walk would do.

Measure Your Neighborhood's Walkability

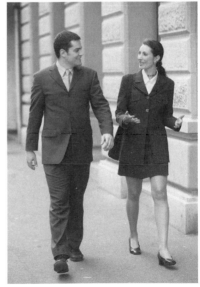

Search the Web (see "Walkable Communities" under Resources) or copy the walkability checklist at the end of the Resource section. Hand them out to neighbors, friends, and family, and have them fill one out on a typical walk. Then collect them and look for common problem areas. Share your findings with city hall and the department of public works, then start to advocate for

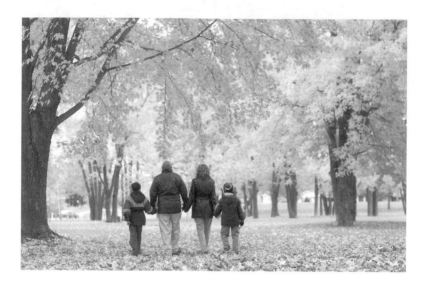

improvements. Many walking facilities are neglected only because no one has asked for help or regular maintenance.

Organize a Walk to School Day

One of the most exciting walking events happening in the United States and around the world (especially England and Canada) is International Walk to School Day. The idea is simple—parents, caregivers, and children are encouraged to walk to school on this one day (usually the first Wednesday in October) to recognize the need for safe, accessible walking routes, and the importance of daily activity for kids. (Children are at the same risks for inactivity as adults in America; childhood obesity rates have skyrocketed in the past 30 years. See the box "Stepping Stone: Stepping Across the Ages" on page 48 in Week Three.) But this is more than a one-day event.

The fundamental idea is to encourage permanent change so children can walk every day, not just on Walk to School Day.

Communities have improved crosswalks, hired crossing guards, launched safety education programs, and repaired sidewalks and pathways as a result of feedback from adults and kids during Walk to School events. Many use walkability checklists so that walkers can catalog opportunities for improvement during their walks.

Start a Walking School Bus

You've had a Walk to School Day, but how do you keep the kids (and adults) walking? By launching a walking school bus, of course. The notion is to create standard routes that children will use to walk to school with adult supervision. As the "bus" walks the route (sometimes participants wear colored hats or scarves), children are picked up along the way. It's not uncommon for the adults to pull a wagon for the children's book bags.

This has the immense advantage of keeping kids walking year-round—"walking buses" have been successful in cold-weather cities such as Chicago and Toronto—while allaying parents' safety

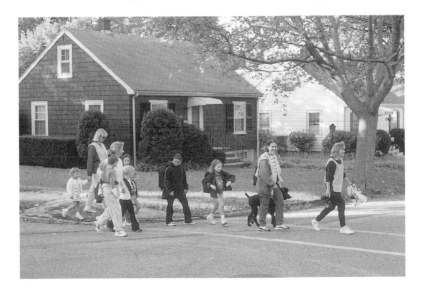

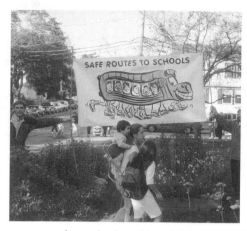

concerns. Children are taught safe pedestrian behaviors, and the environment becomes safer simply because there are more people out and about.

Show Up at Local Governance Meetings

Many of the most important decisions regarding the walkability of your community are made at the local level. How your local planning and zoning board allocates open space, whether it requires sidewalks in new neighborhoods, where schools are built, and the location of commercial centers has a vast impact on whether you can walk as a part of your daily life. You won't often walk to a corner store to buy milk if the "corner store" is 5 miles away, and that's just what happens if developers adhere to most modern zoning codes.

Most codes assume that a separation of uses is good, dating from a time when our industries were filthy and we didn't want their pollution where we lived. But now that the spaces between where we work and live and shop and play are so distant from one another, we are required to go almost everywhere by car. In fact, the U.S. Department of Transportation says that 90 percent or more of all trips are now taken by car! (A terrifying thought given the skyrocketing price of oil.)

You have to speak up if you want that to change. Show up at planning meetings, and demand that new developments have sidewalks and zoning to include corner stores and services within walking distance of homes. Insist that schools be built within the walking distance of as many children as possible. Advocate for the preservation of open space and linear parks with pathways and trails to connect neighborhoods, schools, and commercial areas. Rest assured that your voice will be heard. We've gotten involved in our towns, and been surprised at how few people actually show up and speak up at such public meetings—yet those who do have a substantial influence on the process.

Sell One Car . . . Or All of Them

American families are fast approaching the average of one car for every driver in the house. Of course we *should* be moving in the opposite direction. Getting rid of one car in a two or three-car

PEDOMETER PRO

Claire Tinkerhess:
Buying Steps from Her Employees

Claire Tinkerhess is one businesswoman who puts her money where her mouth is. Tinkerhess, 44, co-owner of Fourth Ave. Birkenstock in Ann Arbor, Michigan, makes the 10- to 15-minute commute to the store on foot, five out of six days a week. She and her husband Paul, who've owned the store for more than 15 years, want their employees to benefit from walking, too, so they pay a bonus of $2 every day an employee chooses not to drive to work—a not-too-shabby $40 a month for a dedicated walker. Claire knows about the health benefits of walking, but as a business owner she sees yet another upside. Walking provides the opportunity to talk to neighbors and other store owners, and thus reinforces community bonds—key to the vitality of any downtown. What's more, her car rarely takes up a parking space that could be used by a customer, and she's conserving oil. Though Claire says it might take a bit more planning to walk to work—she has to watch the clock more closely and think about what she can carry—the hassles are few. Particularly if you're wearing footwear that keeps you comfortable. Her recommendation? Why, Birkies, of course.

STEPPING STONE

10 Benefits of a More Walkable Community

Just in case you have any doubt that it's worth your time, here are 10 quick reasons you need to build or move to a more walkable community (all based on research):

1. **Health.** The easy one—go somewhere it's safer and more inviting to walk and you'll collect more steps and live a longer, healthier life. Enough said on that.

2. **Economics.** Local businesses do better when residents walk and shop locally, rather than driving to distant malls.

3. **Housing values.** Your home will be worth more in a safer, more walkable community. Plus, businesses will want to locate there—it will be easier to keep employees, and they'll be healthier.

4. **Safety.** Police officers put it thusly: Having more eyes on the street is a tremendous deterrent to crime. So more people out walking makes for safer neighborhoods.

5. **Cleaner air.** Cars create vast amounts of air pollution and are a huge contributor to the gases that cause global warming.

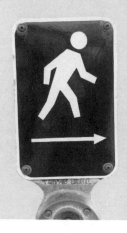

household will save you a bunch of cash (research says operating a car costs $6,500 to $8,000 a year including purchase, debt service, and maintenance—and that doesn't include any environmental and health impacts). But what losing one car really does is help you break the habit of walking out the door and assuming you're always driving to wherever you're going. You'll actually have to ask yourself, *Do I really need the car right now, or can I leave it?*— for your spouse, roommate, kids, and so on.

The ultimate example is going car-free. Car-sharing programs are growing fast in cities large and small. You can register online

6. **Cleaner water.** The oils, fluids, and pulverized tire dust from cars run off the roads and into the surface water in your community. That alone is enough reason to drive less and get more steps.

7. **Less congestion.** Every time someone walks, it means there's one less car on the road. With research showing that you can't dodge congestion simply by widening highways, we should be building more steps, not more lanes.

8. **Quieter streets.** We've become accustomed to the roar of the automobile, instead of the ring of the bicycle bell. We should be able to walk and ride in neighborhoods!

9. **Less dependence on foreign oil.** With $100 a barrel looming, you can be sure that we won't be able to rely on oil imports indefinitely. We desperately need to remake walking and bicycling as central modes of transportation and help break America's addiction to fossil fuels.

10. **Quality of life.** Walk more and you and your children will know your neighbors, and your neighbors will know you. See them often, and you'll look out for each other the way we all used to. And your children will feel like part of a community. Don't doubt that it's possible—add steps and see for yourself!

(e.g., flexcar.com or zipcar.com) and use a "neighborhood" car whenever you need it, but share the fixed costs with others so you don't pay for all the time it's sitting idle.

Talk to Candidates, Write to Congress, Vote

Federal legislation and state budgets can have a huge impact on you as a walker. Recent federal transportation budgets earmark a small fraction of their funds specifically for bicycle, pedestrian, and transit programs and facilities. Still, since the total budgets are hundreds of *billions* of dollars over several years, that leaves hundreds

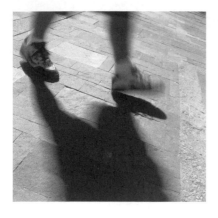

of millions for use by each state for bicycle and pedestrian trails, safety improvements, transit systems, and more.

We must all be vocal advocates for two things: ensuring that those dollars are put to use to benefit pedestrians and bicyclists within our states; and urging that this allocation of our collected tax dollars constantly be increased. It's clear that simply building more roads is not going to solve our congestion, pollution, or energy consumption problems, and it doesn't seem to help our public health, either. Eventually, however, having a lot more Americans walking and biking to the store or work could make a difference on these pressing issues. Let your national and state legislators know you don't want pedestrians to be the "forgotten transportation mode"!

Look for a New House—Live Where You Can Walk!

If you're really ready to take the plunge, then why not move to a community where you can walk more and drive less? There really are places where 9 out of 10 times when you come out the front door to go somewhere, you don't have to start the car—you can simply walk or bicycle where you want to go.

Sound crazy? Well, think for a moment about some of the most desirable cities and towns in America—places that regularly rank high on published lists of America's most livable communities. (Take a look at www.walkable com for some current listings or check our our sampling at the end of the Resources section.) One of the universal elements in these places—from Portland, Maine, to Portland, Oregon, and from Chicago, Illinois, to Austin,

The first week, get your new baseline. Don't change your life, just figure out your daily step average. In Week Two, try to work your steps back up toward your goal. If you've dropped off less than 20 percent, then you can try to get it back all at once. Then in the third week, just make sure you can maintain your 10,000-step (or higher) average.

But if you've dropped off more than 20 percent, don't rush back to 10,000. Work back methodically, adding 10 to 20 percent a week, and rebuild the habits that keep your step totals high.

Texas—is that they are built on a human scale, and they invite you to be out and about on foot. Even big cities such as Seattle, San Francisco, Boston, and Washington, DC, have boulevards and landmarks, parks and pathways that encourage rather than discourage walking. The same holds true for the places we choose to go on vacation, from Nantucket to Santa Fe—one reason we go is because we can walk around there and enjoy it!

The more we preserve and inhabit places that are highly walkable, the more we persuade developers, chambers of commerce, and elected officials to consider this in their future town planning and development. So not only do you make your own life more walkable, but you make a strong statement by your choice as well.

Be a Role Model—Go for a Walk

And so we end where we began—urging you to simply head out the door and go for a walk. Because that is truly what it's all about. When you walk, you improve yourself. But you also improve your community. By your mere presence outside, enjoying one of life's simplest and healthiest activities, you invite others to join you. You change the landscape simply by being there, suggesting to others

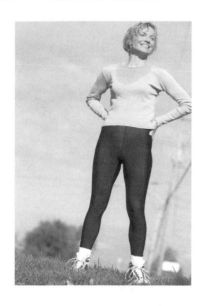

that maybe it is worth heading out and taking a walk. Which, of course, is something you already know.

Week Six Program

Needless to say, if you're below your goal of 10,000 steps a day, continue trying to boost your daily average. There's no crime in taking your time getting there—we've known people who take six months or more to figure out how to build enough steps into their days to consistently average 70,000 steps a week. So just keep chipping away, working to add steps to your routine and making progress toward the goal.

But the big question is this: What are you going to do to make your new, higher step total permanent, whatever that total is? Not just permanent when you remember to wear your pedometer or to check your daily tally. Permanent as in it's the way you think all the time. Permanent as in, "Hey, it's only a 15-minute walk to the theater and we've got 35 minutes before the movie; let's walk." And it's you who's making the suggestion, not your fitness fanatic brother-in-law.

Certainly the first step is to constantly keep reinforcing this as a way of thinking—*Whenever I can, I try to take more steps.* But the real question this week is, are you ready to take a bigger leap? As you've felt the benefits of a healthier lifestyle in just five weeks, have you realized that it's worth keeping it up? You're probably sleeping better, may have lost some weight, and most likely have

STEPS TO SUCCESS

Don't Give That Pedometer Away!

Sure, loan it to your friends if you want, and encourage them to follow this six-week program. But then tell them to get their own pedometers (or be a kind soul and buy each of them one as a congratulatory gift on their success). Why this sudden bout of possessiveness? Because you're going to need your pedometer again, trust us, even if you don't keep wearing it all the time right now. You may be hitting 10,000 steps now or any day now, but there are plenty of ways you can lose ground. Here's just a partial list of the kinds of events that will disrupt a step-full life:

- Starting college.
- Graduating from college.
- Getting married.
- Getting pregnant.
- Having kids.
- Having twins.
- Getting a job.
- Getting fired.
- Getting a new job.
- Getting sick.
- Moving to a new town.
- Having a family member move in.
- Winning the lottery.

You get the idea. All of these disruptions of life and scores of others are enough to throw off your schedule and have you struggling to get 10,000 steps a day. So if any of these happen, or just whenever you sense your steps are slipping, that's the time for a three-week minimum booster program.

greater energy. It's all there for you. This week, make the decision to make the change permanent. Recruit the important people in your life, and make whatever changes are necessary to keep your step-friendly lifestyle. It will be the most important step you take.

PEDOMETER PRO

Steve Turns Back the Clock with a Pedometer

Steve Thompson from Dover, New Hampshire, now 50, was a model of success and living the American dream. He'd been in corporate marketing for 18 years, was making plenty of money, and living with his family in a lovely town. But it was tough—high stress, tight deadlines, a frantic schedule, incessant travel, plus all the necessities of regular life from kids' sports to changing the oil in the car to house repairs.

Steve had been active as a young man, doing yoga, swimming, lifeguarding, and playing sports; in college he was a lean, fit 185 pounds on a 6-foot, 2-inch frame. But that had slowly disappeared with the demands of being a grown-up. Says Steve, "You'd just add five pounds a year, over 10, 15 years. Then all of a sudden you get to 50 and you're 75 pounds overweight." He found the mental exhaustion of corporate life was insidious—instead of coming home and jumping on his bike, he'd open a beer. "You become programmed into habits that are less active. You no longer think about yourself, and think only about everything you've got to do." For years his doctor had warned him that his cholesterol and blood pressure were out of control and he had to lose weight. But Steve thought, *My doctor is fatter than me—why should I listen to this guy?* So he found himself on blood pressure medication and statins for the cholesterol.

Unfortunately, as in so many stories we hear, for Steve it took a major event to recognize what was happening. When Steve was 48 his brother, then 53, had a massive heart attack necessitating a quintuple bypass. His brother checked in at 360 pounds; Steve tipped the scales at 270 and remembers joking with the doctor while visiting his brother, "Well, should I make my reservations *now*?"

They laughed, but Steve got to thinking it was more truth than fiction. He recalls realizing, *I'm going down the wrong path. I need to make a complete reversal, and head in the opposite direction again.* He did it by asking a few simple questions: *When was I happiest in my life? When was I healthiest? When did I have the most energy?* And he took two simple measures to get back there: He got on a balanced diet loaded with whole foods and devoid of refined sugars, and he got a pedometer and started taking 10,000 steps a day, every day.

He went online to find information and a formal program, but still found it plenty challenging: Bad days at work left him with only 2,500 to 3,000 steps, requiring a walk of 7,000 steps at night. He found the pedometer a critically valuable tool: "On really low days I'd think, *Well, crud, I've got to make up my steps at the end of the day.* So you start making concerted effort *during* the day. I'd actually go to the bathroom on purpose to add steps. I'd walk to someone's office instead of call them up. At lunch I'd do a quick walk around the building—I'd ask people to walk with me, even just 15 minutes. You begin thinking ahead and gauging what you have to do to get your 10,000 steps."

His wife, Beth, joined him on many walks and he persevered, walking outdoors even through the worst of New Hampshire's winter. Eventually, he decided that the constant sitting—endless meetings, computer and phone time, even eating at his desk—had to stop. He left his job to start consulting and building his own business, schedule, and lifestyle. And he realized the rewards were vast.

"You find that with every pound you lose on the way back, you peel away another layer of emotional damage, and your self-esteem and self-image start to return," says Steve. One of his real signs of success? "Even your vanity starts to come back. You flex your arms in the mirror and you can say, *Hey, not too bad.*"

But here's the big payoff: Not only did he lose 75 pounds, but in nine months Steve went from having a near-certain date with the cardiac surgeon to getting off both his drugs. And Beth feels he's turned back into the man she married, with a true joy for living. He's playing tennis, doing yoga, even meditating, and he credits the 10,000 steps of daily walking with helping to open all those doors.

Steve offers a warning: "Your current friends might not recognize you as you peel off the pounds. But I saw a buddy from 20 years ago who knew me instantly—proving that I really had moved myself backward in time." It was just as he'd hoped. And lest you think he's keeping the secret to himself, Steve's now got an informal group of more than 20 friends who are on the 10,000-step-a-day plan and healthy-eating kick along with him. Maybe you can follow his lead, and invite a friend on your next walk.

Week Six Step Log

Number of steps	Anything special today?
Monday	
Tuesday	
Wednesday	
Thursday	
Friday	
Saturday	
Sunday	
Week Total	

Daily average: _____
(total steps for the week divided by 7)

Daily goal for next week: _____
(daily average x 1.2, for a 20% increase)

11 Most Frequently Asked Questions

For easy reference, we've compiled what we have found to be the most common burning questions about pedometer walking. If you need more information on any one topic, just follow the page reference and read on. Use these to help get family, friends, and strangers hooked on using a pedometer!

1. What is a pedometer?

A pedometer is a pager-sized device that clips on to your belt or waistband and counts the number of steps you take. When your hip swings, an interior arm swings, too, causing a step to register on the display panel or counter (see "How Pedometers Work," page 3).

2. Where do I get a pedometer?

Check sporting goods and specialty athletic retailers such as running or outdoor gear stores, or look online (see "Pedometer Vendors" in the Resources section).

3. What kind should I get and how much will it cost?

Expect to pay $15 to $30, and look for a simple digital step counter with a numerical LCD readout and a single button to reset the step count to zero. Among the most accurate in research tests were Digi-Walkers (see "Pedometer Vendors" in the Resources section); their steps-only version costs about $20. Pricier models also estimate distance covered and calories burned, but those features aren't necessary. Also key: a sturdy clip and a small safety cord that you can pass through a belt loop or clip to your waistband.

4. How do I wear a pedometer? How do I know it's working right?

Clip the pedometer to your waistband on the front of your waist, in line with one knee. Make sure the pedometer face is perpendicular to the ground—it shouldn't twist left or right, or lean forward or back. (If this is a problem, see "How to Wear a Pedometer" on page 7.) Reset the pedometer to zero, and walk around while you count the steps of both feet until you hit 50. Your count and the pedometer's should be within five steps.

5. When should I wear the pedometer?

Our concept is to measure all of your activity, not just formal exercise, so wear the pedometer all day, every day, unless you're swimming, showering, or naked. Put it on when you get up in the morning, take if off when you climb into bed, write down the total steps, and then reset the pedometer to zero for the next day.

6. What activities count toward my step total? What about bike riding?

Just about anything that moves your hips will register steps on your pedometer. Walking, running, climbing stairs, playing sports such as basketball, tennis, or soccer, and fitness activities such as aerobics classes and workouts on treadmills and stair climbers all contribute. Biking is another story. Pedometers can't measure this hip motion accurately, but if you tie or securely clip the pedometer to the shoelace of one foot, it will count pedal strokes, which is roughly equivalent to counting steps (see page 66 for typical steps).

7. What should my daily step goal be?

Here are three rough targets to aim for. Keep in mind that your lifestyle, diet, and physiology may mean you have to adjust up or down to reach your goal (see page 47 for details).

1. For weight control and a healthier heart, aim for at least 10,000 steps per day.
2. For long-term health plus a more noticeable weight loss (more steps burn more calories), aim for 12,000 to 15,000 steps per day.
3. To boost aerobic fitness (heart and lung strength), make sure that 3,000 of your daily steps are at a fast pace several days a week.

8. How far is 10,000 steps, anyway?

A rough rule of thumb is that 2,000 steps equals a mile, making 10,000 steps about 5 miles. But taller walkers will take fewer steps per mile, and shorter ones will take more. Take a stroll around the local one-quarter-mile track to determine about how many steps you take in a mile, but keep your focus on increasing your daily step totals, not covering a certain distance (see page 28).

9. How do I improve my daily step total?

First, find ways to weave more walking into everyday life—take the stairs, take an extra lap at the mall before you shop. You've heard it before, but now you can actually measure these additions, because you have a pedometer. Second, add structured step boost-ers (think daily morning walk and bimonthly hike, page 71). A more extreme strategy: Move to a location where work and errands are within walking distance, or to a neighborhood that offers safe sidewalks, walking trails, and bike paths (page 104). In other words, make more steps part of every single day.

10. Can my pedometer estimate the distance I walk? Or the calories I burn?

By calibrating your pedometer, you can get a fair estimate of the distance you cover in a given walk, because people's strides tend to be consistent at a given speed. To measure your stride length for a pedometer that measures distance: Use the pedometer to count your steps for exactly one trip around the inside lane of a one-quarter-mile track. Divide 1,320 feet (a quarter mile) by the num-ber of steps you took to calculate your stride length, and enter that in the pedometer according to the instructions (page 31).

As for calorie burn, pedometer estimates aren't reliable—there are too many factors at play for this to be accurate (page 33).

11. What if I get stuck in a rut and can't add any more steps to my days?

If you're using all the tools from Weeks One through Five and find yourself more active, but not enough to satisfy your goals, fear not. Dig into Week Six for fresh strategies to help you take it up a notch and create a truly active lifestyle.

Resources

Events: Walking Events, Organizers, and Information

American Diabetes Association's Team Diabetes Walks: Marathon
training program. 888-342-2383; www.walk.diabetes.org.

American Heart Association (AHA): American Heart Walk.
800-AHA-USA1 (800-242-8721); www.americanheart.org.

American Volksport Association (AVA): AVA's 500 clubs organize
more than 3,000 events per year nationwide. 800-830-WALK
(800-830-9255); www.ava.org.

Arthritis Foundation's Joints in Motion Event: Marathon training
program. 800-960-7682; www.arthritis.org.

Avon's 3-Day Breast Cancer Walks: 60-mile group walks including
food, tent accommodations, and entertainment. 866-668-WALK
(866-668-9255); www.avoncrusade.com.

Leukemia Society of America Marathons: Marathon training program.
800-482-TEAM (800-482-8326); www.teamintraining.org.

March of Dimes WalkAmerica: Events from 5 to 20 kilometers
(approximately 12 miles). 800-525-WALK (800-525-9255);
www.modimes.org.

MS Walk: Walks from 3 to 12 miles; 800-FIGHT-MS (800-344-4867); www.nmss.org.

Race for the Cure: The largest series of 5K and 1-mile run/fitness walks in the nation. 888-603-RACE (888-603-7223); www.raceforthecure.com.

Hiking Information

American Hiking Society: A national hiking and trail advocacy organization, which can help you get in touch with a club in your area. 301-565-6704; www.americanhiking.org.

Appalachian Mountain Club: America's oldest conservation and recreation organization, based in the Northeast. The AMC teaches skills, operates lodges, fixes trails, publishes guides, and works on conservation issues. To join a local chapter or get more information, contact 617-523-0636 or www.outdoors.org.

Sierra Club: This well-known environmental organization provides information on current environmental issues, teaches conservation skills, and sponsors 330 national and international outings per year. For more information, call the national office at 415-977-5500 or visit www.sierraclub.org.

Nordic Walking (walking poles)

Exel: 802-524-4770; www.nordicwalker.com.
Exerstrider: 800-554-0989; www.exerstrider.com.
Leki: 716-683-1022; www.leki.com.
Swix: 978-657-4820; www.swixnordicwalking.us/.

Pedometer Programs

AARP Step Up to Better Health program:www.aarp.org/health/fitness/ walking; then click on "Step Up to Better Health."
Register online for this 10-week pedometer-based walking promotion. Reduced-price pedometers are available to AARP members, and you can

log your steps on the Web site to see your progress virtually charted along a major American pathway, such as the Appalachian Trail.

America on the Move: www.americaonthemove.org.
An innovative online pedometer program developed by Dr. James Hill at the Center for Human Nutrition at the University of Colorado Health Sciences Center in Denver. The goal is for participants to increase their activity by 2,000 steps per day, and to decrease consumption by 100 Calories per day. Dr. Hill believes that this amount of exercise, while probably not enough to result in weight loss, can prevent the weight gain associated with "creeping obesity." In an article published in *Science*, Hill notes that American adults gain an average of 1.8 pounds per year. He feels that most Americans could halt creeping weight gain by doing even a little extra activity every day. "The whole idea is, if we can get people more active, we can greatly improve health and reduce weight gain," says Hill.

President's Council on Physical Fitness and Sports: www.fitness.gov.
The President's Council Active Lifestyle program, begun in 2002, encourages people to get active by doing 30 minutes of physical activity a day, five days per week, for at least six weeks. Participants are encouraged to track their activity online, but they can also do so using a paper version of the form. If you enjoy walking or jogging, you're encouraged to use a pedometer to log your steps, instead of time. The step goals vary with age: 10,000 steps per day for adults; 11,000 steps per day for girls age 6 through 17; and 13,000 steps for boys 6 through 17. Once you've earned your Presidential Active Lifestyle Award, you can send away for merchandise (patches, T-shirts, magnets, bumper stickers).

www.pedometers.com.
A Web site with performance reviews and rankings of pedometers and more technical information than you'd ever want about how the things actually work.

Health Partners' 10,000 Steps® Program: www.10k-steps.com
Health Partners, a nonprofit HMO based in Minnesota, sponsors a 10,000 steps program. You can subscribe to a mail-based or Internet version of the program and receive a high quality Digi-Walker pedometer. They'll

send you regular mailings, allow you to log your steps online, and answer your questions over the phone.

Walkingworks: www.walkingworks.com.
Blue Cross/Blue Shield sponsors a WalkingWorks program to encourage Americans to get active. As one of the nation's largest health insurance providers, BCBS has a vested interest in keeping its members healthy and fit. Pedometers can be purchased at a very low price ($4.95 as of this book's printing), and participants are encouraged to strive for 10,000 steps or 30 minutes of activity per day, on five or more days a week. To avoid injury, BCBS recommends that if you are not already a walker, you should establish a baseline over seven days to see how active you are. (Sounds good to us.) It then urges modest increases in daily steps over the following weeks.

Pedometer Vendors

Accusplit
 www.accusplit.com
 2290A Ringwood Avenue
 Silicon Valley (San Jose), CA 95131

 For Sales Assistance
 Phone: 800-935-1996
 Fax: 408-432-0316
 International calls: 408-432-8228, ext.4
 E-mail: sales@accusplit.com

 For Postsale Assistance
 Phone: 800-965-2008
 Fax: 408-432-0316
 E-mail: support@accusplit.com

Bodytronics
 www.bodytronics.com
 TKO Enterprises, Inc.
 220 Etowah Trace
 Fayetteville, GA 30214

Phone: 678-817-5789
Fax: 678-817-5830
E-mail: support2@bodytronics.com

New Lifestyles, Inc.
www.new-lifestyles.com
www.digiwalker.com
5201 NE Maybrook Road
Lee's Summit, MO 64064
Order line: 888-748-5377
Customer service: 816-373-9969
Fax: 816-373-9929
E-mail: info@new-lifestyles.com

Optimal Health Products
www.optimalhealthproducts.com
4900 Broadway, Suite 200
San Antonio, TX 78209
Phone: 888-339-2067

Step Into Health
www.stepintohealth.com
2314 Route 59, #190
Plainfield, IL 60544
Phone: 815-609-9733
Fax: 815-609-9134
E-mail: customercare@stepintohealth.com

Walk4Life
www.walk4life.com
12137 Rhea Drive, Unit B
Plainfield, IL 60544
Phone: 888-422-1806 or 815-439-2340
Fax: 815-439-2414
Sales: sales@walk4life.com
Customer service: customerservice@walk4life.com

Features of Some Common Pedometer Models

Company	Model	Step-Count Accuracy	Functions*	Approx. Cost
New Lifestyles	NL-2000	Excellent	S, C, 7-day M	$50
Yamax	SW-200**	Excellent	S	$25
Yamax	SW-701**	Excellent	S, D, C	$30
Colorado On the Move	X120	Very good	S	$25
Yamax	Skeletone	Very good	S	$15
Walk4Life	LS 2525	Very good	S, D, C	$29
Omron	HJ-105	Good	S, D, C	$27
Freestyle	Pacer Pro	Fair	S, D, C	$20
Accusplit	Alliance1510	Fair	S, D, C	$20
Sportline	345	Fair	S, D, C	$30
Sportline	330	Poor	S	$13
Oregon Scientific	PE316CA	Poor	S, D, C	$20

*Functions: S = steps, D = distance, C = calories, M = memory
**Yamax SW series pedometers are also sold under the names New Lifestyles Digi-Walker, Accusplit Eagle, and Walk4Life Life Stepper.

Racewalking

North American Racewalking Foundation: More racewalking information, tips, and contacts than you'll ever want. www.philsport.com/narf/; 626-795-3243.

Racewalk.com: A comprehensive site with resources, books, and merchandise on racewalking. www.racewalk.com.

USA Track and Field: The national governing body for track and field and racewalking in the United States. To find your regional track and field office and connect with local racewalking leads, contact the national office: 317-261-0500; www.usatf.org/groups/racewalking.

Walkable Communities

Select resources to help in creating a more livable, walkable, step-friendly community.

Active Living by Design program of the Robert Wood Johnson Foundation, Chapel Hill, North Carolina: An extensive online research bibliography and lots of links to further resources. www.activelivingbydesign.org; 919-843-2523.

Association of Pedestrian and Bicycle Professionals (APBP): An organization of professionals in transportation planning and engineering with expertise in creating more walkable, bicycle-friendly settings. www.apbp.org.

AmericaWalks, Boston, Massachusetts: A coalition of more than 50 local and regional pedestrian advocacy groups nationwide, providing technical resources, support, and training opportunities. 617-367-1170; www.americawalks.org.

Bikes Belong Coalition, Ltd., Brookline, Massachusetts: A coalition of bicycle industry supporters working to create more livable and bicycle-safe communities. www.bikesbelong.org.

Centers for Disease Control and Prevention: A Web site with lots of current data on health and physical activity, and promotional resources. www.cdc.gov/nccdphp/dnpa.

League of American Bicyclists, Washington, DC: A national advocacy group advancing the Bike Friendly Communities program; it also provides training and certification for (and access to) bicycle safety instructors. 202-822-1333; www.bikeleague.org.

Local Government Commission, Sacramento, California: A huge library of practical planning and transportation guides for elected officials and community leaders, including the very accessible guide *Real Towns.* 916-448-1198; www.lgc.org.

National Center for Bicycling and Walking, Washington, DC: A national advocacy organization that provides Walkable Community Workshops to communities and regions, and organizes the biennial Pro Walk/Pro Bike conference. 301-656-4220; www.bikewalk.org.

Pedestrian and Bicycle Information Center, Chapel Hill, North Carolina: Technical support for communities, including walkability and bikeability checklists and bicycle and pedestrian facility design guides. Be sure to check out the online image library. 877-WALK-BIKE; www.walkinginfo.org; www.bicyclinginfo.org.

Rails-to-Trails Conservancy, Washington, DC: Great help for trails advocates, including research supporting the proven benefits of trails. 202-331-9696; www.railtrails.org.

Rivers and Trails Conservation Assistance: A program of the National Park Service that provides technical support to communities working to build pathways, greenways, and water trails. Fax: 202-354-6900; www.ncrc.nps.gov/rtca.

Surface Transportation Policy Project, Washington, DC: This project publishes numerous reports loaded with pedestrian travel and safety data; great to back up local advocacy efforts. 202-466-2636; www.transact.org.

Walk a Child to School Day: Tons of information on putting on a Walk to School event and finding more information. United States: www.walktoschool.org.

Walkable Communities, Inc.: The nonprofit creation of Dan Burden, one of the nation's leading experts and consultants on creating more livable, pedestrian-friendly communities. 866-347-2734; www.walkable.org.

Some of America's Most Walkable Communities

Author Mark Fenton travels the country working with transportation, planning, and health agencies and advocates as they strive to create safer and more inviting communities for walking. Here's his list of some of America's most walkable places. By no means comprehensive, this is just a sampling of cities and towns across the country benefiting from current efforts to get people to celebrate the joy of walking.

Large cities

Boston, Massachusetts. Lots of pre-automobile history—nearly 400 years' worth—and growth constrained by water on three sides

assured that at its inception Boston took on a compact, magnifi-
cently walkable form. Walk the Freedom Trail and explore Boston
Common, but don't drive. Use the "T" (the oldest subway system in
the nation) to get around; you probably won't be able to find a place
to "pahk the cah" anyway.

Chicago, Illinois. A little wind doesn't keep droves of Chicagoans away
from the Lakeshore Path; it's ideal for walking, cycling, and in-line
skating, and especially people-watching. A traditional grid and a fine
transit system make Chicago eminently walkable, and great architecture and statuary (and, frankly, food) make it worth exploring on foot.

Minneapolis, Minnesota. This is a city laced with trails and bike lanes,
many of which connect neighborhoods and the green space sur-
rounding innumerable lakes. Car-free Nicolette Boulevard, a light
rail system (thanks to former Governor Jesse Ventura), and lots of
residential redevelopment further boost its walkable appeal. Stroll
the Stone Arch Bridge across the Mississippi River, preserved only
for bike, pedestrian, and trolley traffic.

New York, New York. This city may never sleep, but it sure does walk a
lot. Every block is a walker's delight to explore—you never know
what type of restaurant, shop, or street vendor you'll stumble on
next—but New York's also building a world-class greenway system,
beginning with non-motorized pathways which will soon circle all
of Manhattan and connect into the other boroughs. Set aside time
for aimless rambling through Central Park, the masterpiece of the
father of landscape architecture, Frederick Law Olmstead.

Portland, Oregon. A pedestrianized downtown, a growing network of
bike lanes and pathways, and mixed-use development that encourages neighborhoods where life, work, and play are all within walking distance are all the results of two decades' worth of policy
efforts. Walk the waterfront trails along the Willamette River,
including the bridges and amazing floating walkway.

San Francisco, California. The hills only enhance the appeal of
strolling the colorful neighborhoods of the City by the Bay. Mother
Nature made a cataclysmic improvement to the pedestrian network,
crumbling the elevated Embarcadero Freeway in a 1989 earthquake.
Take an amble along the rebuilt surface boulevard (with light rail

service and great bike and walk connectivity) along the waterfront all the way to the Presidio—a former military base and now beautiful urban park—and then out onto the Golden Gate Bridge.

Seattle, Washington. You feel the outdoor ethic of the Pacific Northwest as you circle Green Lake or wander the pedestrian friendly neighborhoods such as Queen Ann, Capitol Hill, and downtown. The Burke-Gilman Trail, 30 years old, 30 miles long and still growing, is a non-motorized spine through the city that sets the standard for urban trails nationwide. Walk onto the Puget Sound ferries, and then explore the island destinations on foot.

Washington, DC. Parisian planner Pierre Charles L'Enfant laid out the city as an easily navigated grid with angled boulevards connecting grand civic buildings and creating scores of inviting public circles and pocket parks. Add a great subway system, still-growing trail network, and more national monuments than you can shake a stick at, and you've got a national capitol a pedestrian can be proud of. Wander from the National Mall to Georgetown, then out a ways along the C&O Canal tow path trail.

These large cities are so well equipped for walking (and have such great transit) that it's not even worth driving or renting a car there. Go pure pedestrian!

Medium-sized cities

Arlington, Virginia. Transit-oriented development makes it easy to live without a car in this Washington, DC, suburb.

Austin, Texas. Riverfront trails and some stunning pathway bridges invite exploration by bike and on foot.

Boulder, Colorado. One of America's first car-free zones, Pearl Street Mall, is still one of the best, along with great trails, transit, and pedestrian boulevards.

Burlington, Vermont. Walk the waterfront trail along Lake Champlain, and explore the downtown pedestrian zone.

Cambridge, Massachusetts. A network of bike lanes, the Charles River waterfront trail, and great walkable neighborhoods.

Chattanooga, Tennessee. Saving the bridge at Walnut Street for bicyclists and pedestrians stimulated a riverfront trail system and downtown comeback.

Davis, California. A conscious effort begun 30 years ago to keep the city from being overrun by cars has made this America's bicycling capitol!

Indianapolis, Indiana. The Monon Trail—the centerpiece of a growing trail system—snakes from rejuvenated downtown neighborhoods to the suburbs.

Lincoln, Nebraska. A growing trail system and traditional downtown grid boost walking in this university town.

Madison, Wisconsin. State Street is always full of bikes and pedestrians, as are the trails around the city's lakes.

Mt. Lebanon, Pennsylvania. So committed to walkable neighborhood schools that no child is bussed to school.

Portland, Maine. Great waterfront walking defines this inviting New England port city, including the inner harbor area.

Santa Barbara, California. Walk the oceanfront trail to kayak, surf, find outdoor dining, or just to walk; then bike up to the historic mission.

West Palm Beach, Florida. A model of urban redevelopment that used walkability as a central tenet of the economic rebirth.

Smaller cities and towns
(just a sampling of the hundreds across the United States!)

Alexandria, Virginia
Annapolis, Maryland
Arcata, California
Brockport, New York
Charleston, South Carolina
Chautauqua, New York
Crested Butte, Colorado
Dunedin, Florida
Exeter, New Hampshire
Glenwood Springs, Colorado
Jackson, Wyoming
Kirkland, Washington

Livingston, Montana
Portsmouth, New Hampshire
Saratoga Springs, New York
Savannah, Georgia
Traverse City, Michigan
Xenia, Ohio

Neighborhood Walkability Checklist

(Adapted from the checklist of the Partnership for a Walkable America;
www.walkinginfo.org)

Take this checklist on a typical walk (to a friend's house, your child's day-
care, the corner store) and share copies with friends. Note things that
might discourage you (and a child) from walking regularly and their locations. Score each from 1 to 6; compare notes with others to identify the
biggest problems. Then talk to public officials and set priorities for making improvements.

1. Did you have room to walk?   **Score:** _____

(6=room for 2 or 3 people; 1=barely enough for 1)

If no, note specific problems, such as no sidewalks
or broken ones; sidewalks blocked with poles, signs,
or dumpsters; no paths or trails; no shoulders.

Comments, locations: _____

_____

2. Was it easy to cross streets?   **Score:** _____

(6=no problem; 1=it took forever and was scary)

If no, note specific problems, such as roads too wide
to get across; signals made for long waits, or didn't
give enough crossing time; striped crosswalks or traffic signals are lacking; parked cars, trees or other
things blocked view of traffic; curb ramps are lacking.

Comments, locations: _____

_____

3. Was traffic a problem?   **Score:** _____

(6=didn't notice it; 1=lots of cars, too fast, too close)

If yes, note specific problems, such as too many
cars, or traffic was too fast; drivers backed out of
driveways without looking; drivers did not yield to

pedestrians, but turned toward people crossing side streets; drivers drove too fast, sped up to get through traffic lights, stopped in or blocked crosswalks.

Comments, locations: _____

_____

4. Did you feel safe?   Score: _____
(6=I'd walk alone anytime; 1=scary, even with others, in daylight)

If no, note specific problems, such as suspicious activity or people; no apparent houses, stores, or other places to go in case of trouble; no public telephones; too dark; too few other pedestrians; too little activity on the street.

Comments, locations: _____

_____

5. Was it a pleasant place to walk?   Score: _____
(6=I'd love to go back; 1=no reason to be there)

If no, note specific problems, such as more grass, flowers, or trees, water fountains, shade, benches should be added; too dark, dirty; no art, natural, architectural, or historic features; few desirable destinations (stores, restaurants, a library, post office, schools, bus or subway stops) along the way.

Comments, locations: _____

_____

Check your score:
26–30:   Terrific. You live in a great walking community.
21–25:   Good. But focus on trouble spots.
16–20:   Fair. Get your neighbors and elected officials involved immediately.
15 or less: Call out the National Guard—it's no fun walking there, and it needs work.

Making the World More Walkable

If your walking route scored poorly, then take action. Share your findings with elected officials (for example, the mayor's office or city council) and public services. Start with the department of public works, transportation, and police departments. Let them—and the media—know about specific trouble spots. Also, get out and fix what you can. Here are some simple things you can do; urge family and friends to join your efforts:

Do it yourself.

- Select better, safer routes to walk if necessary. But that's not enough!
- Trim hedges or trees that block sidewalks or the view at a crosswalk.
- Plant beautifying trees and flowers if you have property abutting sidewalks or trails.
- Organize a neighborhood clean-up day, or just take a bag and pick up trash on your normal walking routes. Always clear your sidewalk of snow or debris.
- Be a considerate driver. Set an example: drive at safe speeds in neighborhoods, let pedestrians cross at intersections, don't stop in crosswalks.
- Notify the animal control officer of problem animals, and the police of suspicious activity. Report street or signal lights that are out to the department of public works.

Change your community.

- Speak up at governance and planning meetings. Demand bicycle and pedestrian friendly planning, engineering, and policies. For detailed information, contact:
- Pedestrian and Bicycle Information Center: www.pedbikeinfo.org.
- National Center for Bicycling and Walking: www.bikewalk.org.
- The RWJF Active Living by Design Program: www.activeliving bydesign.org.

Build a trail.

- Learn how trails improve health: www.cdc.gov/nccdphp/dnpa /physical/trails.htm
- Get a railroad right-of-way turned into a trail; contact the Rails-to-Trails Conservancy for assistance at: www.railtrails.org.

Get kids walking to school.

- Hold a Walk to School Day event; www.walktoschool.org.
- Set up a walking school bus and a full safe-routes-to-school program: www.walkinginfo.org.

Be a role model by walking somewhere every day.

Encourage others by your actions. For a detailed resource list, and comprehensive information on starting or maintaining a walking program, take a look at *The Complete Guide to Walking for Health, Weight Loss, and Fitness* by Mark Fenton (The Lyons Press, 2001)

Further Reading and References

Books on Walking and Pedometry

Manpo-Kei: The Art and Science of Step Counting, by Catrine Tudor-Locke. Victoria, BC; Trafford Publishing, 2003. One of the leading pedometer researchers summarizes her insights and experiences in promoting the use of pedometers.

The Complete Guide to Walking for Health, Weight Loss, and Fitness, by Mark Fenton. Guilford, CT: Lyons Press, 2001. A comprehensive information source on America's favorite fitness activity, including a one-year walking program.

Walking Through Pregnancy and Beyond, by Mark and Lisa Fenton and Tracy Teare. Guilford, CT: Lyons Press, 2004. A guide for safe, healthy exercise through the nine months of pregnancy and the year following delivery.

Pedometer Power: 67 Lessons for K–12, by Robert P. Pangrazi, Aaron Beighle, and Cara L. Sidman. Champaign, IL: Human Kinetics, 2004. Three physical educators describe creative uses of pedometers in elementary, middle, and high school settings.

Pedometer Walking: A New Look At Walking, Longevity, Weight Management, and Active Living, by Robert Sweetgall. Advice, insights, and motivational tips from the long-distance guru who has walked across the United States seven times.

Articles and Research

General

Bassett DR, Strath SC. Use of pedometers to assess physical activity. In *Physical Activity Assessments for Health-Related Research,* G Welk, editor. Champaign, IL: Human Kinetics Publishers, 2004.

Sidman C. Count your steps to health and fitness. *American College of Sports Medicine's Health and Fitness Journal* 6(1):13–17, 2002.

Sidman C, Corbin CB, LeMasurier G. Promoting physical activity among sedentary women using pedometers. *Research Quarterly for Exercise and Sport* 75:122–129, 2004.

Tudor-Locke C. Taking steps toward increased physical activity: using pedometers to measure and motivate. *Research Digest* 3(17), June 2002.

Week One

Flegal KM, Carroll MD, Odgen CL., Johnson CL. Prevalence and trends in obesity among U.S. adults, 1999–2000. *Journal of the American Medical Association* 288:1723–1727, 2002.

Ogden CL, Fryar CD, Carroll MD, Flegal KM. Mean body weight, height, and body mass index, United States 1960–2002. *Advance Data from Vital and Health Statistics* 347, October 27, 2004.

Spurlock, M. *Don't Eat This Book: Fast Food and the Super-Sizing of America.* New York: G. P. Putnam's Sons, 2005.

Schlosser, E. *Fast Food Nation: The Dark Side of the All-American Meal.* New York: Houghton Mifflin, 2001.

Critser, G. *Fat Land: How Americans Became the Fattest People in the World.* Boston: Houghton Mifflin, 2003.

Frank LD, Andresen MA, Schmid TL. Obesity relationships with community design, physical activity, and time spent in cars. *American Journal of Preventive Medicine* 27(2):87–96, 2004.

Schoenborn CA, Adams PF, Barnes PM. Body weight status of adults: United States, 1997–1998. *Advance Data from Vital and Health Statistics* 330:1–15, 2002.

Martinez JA, Kearney JM, Kafatos A, Paquet S, Martinez-Gonzalez MA. Variables independently associated with self-reported obesity in the European Union. *Public Health Nutrition* 2:125–133, 1999.

Organization for Economic Cooperation and Development. *Health at a Glance: OECD Indicators 2003*. Paris, France: OECD Publications Service, 2003.

Schneider PL, Crouter SE, Lukajic O, Bassett DR. Accuracy and reliability of 10 pedometers for measuring steps over a 400-m walk. *Medicine and Science in Sports and Exercise* 35:1779–1784, 2003.

Crouter SE, Schneider PL, Karabult M, Bassett DR. Validity of ten electronic pedometers for measuring steps, distance, and kcals during treadmill walking. *Medicine and Science in Sports and Exercise* 35:1455–1460, 2003.

Hatano Y. Use of the pedometer for promoting daily walking exercise. *International Council for Health, Physical Education, and Recreation (ICHPER) Journal* 29(4):4–8, 1993.

Palletta, L. A., and Worth, F., editors. *World Almanac of Presidential Facts*. New York: Pharos, 1993.

Dumbauld, E. *Thomas Jefferson: American Tourist*. Norman: University of Oklahoma Press, 1946.

Nock, A. J. *Jefferson*. New York: Harcourt, Brace, and Co., 1926.

Wilson, D. L., and Standon, L., editors. *Jefferson Abroad*. New York: Modern Library, 1999.

Hellmich N. Get with the 2,000 step program: walk an extra mile, shoo away weight gain. *USA Today*, October 24, 2002, 8D.

Levine JA. Role of nonexercise activity thermogenesis in resistance to fat gain in humans. *Science* 283:212–214, 1999.

Vincent SD, Pangrazi RP, Raustorp A, Tomson LM, Cuddihy TF. Activity levels and body mass index of children in the United States, Sweden, and Australia. *Medicine and Science in Sports and Exercise* 35(8):1367–1373, 2003.

Cardon GM, DeBourdeaudhuij IMM. A pilot study comparing pedometer counts with physical activity minutes in elementary school children. *Medicine and Science in Sports and Exercise* 36(5):S31, 2004.

Rowlands AV, Eston RG, Ingledew DK. Relationships between activity levels, aerobic fitness, and body fat in 8- to 10-yr old children. *Journal of Applied Physiology* 86:1428–1435, 1998.

Wyatt HR, Peters JC, Reed GT, Barry M, and Hill JO. A Colorado statewide survey of walking and its relation to excessive weight gain. *Medicine and Science in Sports and Exercise* 37: 724–730, 2005.

Hakim AA, Curb JD, Petrovich H. Effects of walking on coronary heart disease in elderly men: the Honolulu Heart Program. *Circulation* 100:9–13, 1999.

Lee I-M, Rexrode KM, Cook NR, Manson JE, Buring JE. Physical activity and coronary heart disease in women: is "no pain, no gain" passé? *Journal of the American Medical Association* 285(11):1447–1454, 2001.

International Agency for Research on Cancer. World Health Organization. Overweight and lack of exercise linked to increased cancer risk: a growing problem. www.iarc.fr/index.htmal. Last accessed on August 27, 2005.

Manson JE, Hu FB, Rich-Edwards JW, Colditz GA, Stampfer MJ, Willett WC, et al. A prospective study of walking as compared with vigorous exercise in the prevention of coronary heart disease in women. *New England Journal of Medicine* 341:650–658, 1999.

Holmes MD, Chen WY, Feskanisch D, Kroenke CH, Colditz GA. Physical activity and survival after breast cancer diagnosis. *Journal of the American Medical Association* 293 (20): 2479–2487, 2005.

Moreau KL, DeGarmo R, Langley J, McMahon C, Howley ET, Bassett DR, Thompson DL. Increasing daily walking lowers blood pressure in post-menopausal women. *Medicine and Science in Sports and Exercise* 33:1825–1831, 2001.

Swartz AM, Strath SJ, Bassett DR, Moore JB, Redwine BA, Groer M, Thompson DL. Increasing daily walking improves glucose tolerance in overweight women. *Preventive Medicine* 37:356–362, 2003.

Gibbs-Smith, C. *The Inventions of Leonardo da Vinci.* London: Phaidon Press, 1978.

Breguet, E. *Breguet: Watchmakers Since 1775*. Paris: Alain de Gourcuff, 1997.

Koga S, Baugh RA, Decker W, Minetti AE, Rossiter H, Ward S, Whipp BJ. Paleo-energetics and biomechanics. Symposium presented at the American College of Sports Medicine, 50th Annual Meeting, San Francisco, May 28–31, 2003.

Sequeira MM, Richardson M, Wietlisbach V, Tullen B, Schutz Y. Physical activity assessment using a pedometer and its comparison with a questionnaire in a large population study. *American Journal of Epidemiology* 142:9989–9999, 1995.

McCormack G, Milligan R, Giles-Corti B, Clarkson JP. *Physical Activity Levels of Western Australia Adults 2002: Results from the Adult Physical Activity Survey and Pedometer Study*. Perth, Western Australia: Western Australian Government. www.patf.dpc.wa.gov.au. Last accessed August 9, 2005.

Tudor-Locke C, Ham SA, Macera CA, Ainsworth BE, Kirtland KA, Reis JP, Kimsey CD. Descriptive epidemiology of pedometer-determined physical activity. *Medicine and Science in Sports and Exercise* 36:1567–1573, 2004.

Tudor-Locke C, Myers A. Methodological considerations for researchers and practitioners using pedometers to measure physical (ambulatory) activity. *Research Quarterly for Exercise and Sport* 72:1–12, 2001.

Crouter S, Schneider PL, Bassett DR. Accuracy of pedometers for measuring steps in overweight and obese individuals. *Medicine and Science in Sports and Exercise* 37:S23, 2005.

Week Two

Hill JO, Wyatt HR, Reed GW, Peters JC. Obesity and the environment: where do we go from here? *Science* 299:853–855, 2003.

Dunn AL, Marcus BH, Kampert JB, Garcia ME, Kohl HW, Blair SN. Comparison of lifestyle and structured interventions to increase physical activity and cardiorespiratory fitness: a random trial. *Journal of the American Medical Association* 281:327–334, 1999.

Klem ML, Wing RR, McGuire MT, Seagle HM, Hill JO. A descriptive study of individuals successful at long-term maintenance of substantial weight loss. *American Journal of Clinical Nutrition* 66:239–246, 1997.

U.S. Department of Agriculture and U.S. Department of Health and Human Services. Dietary Guidelines for Americans 2005. www.health.gov/dietaryguidelines/dga2005/document. Last accessed August 9, 2005.

Miyatake N, Nishikawa H, Morishita A, Kunitomi M, Wada J, Suzuki H, et al. Daily walking reduces visceral adipose tissue areas and improves insulin resistance in Japanese obese males. *Diabetes Research and Clinical Practice* 58:101–107, 2002.

Hellmich N. Journey to better fitness starts with 10,000 steps. *USA Today*, 8–9, June 29, 1999.

Uhlman M. Pedometer's popularity taking off. *Philadelphia Inquirer*, A16, October 12, 2002.

Week Three

Tudor-Locke CE, Bassett DR. How many steps are enough? Pedometer-determined physical activity indices. *Sports Medicine* 34:1–8, 2004.

Hatano Y. Prevalence and use of pedometer [article written in Japanese]. *Research Journal of Walking* 1:45–54, 1997.

Hatano Y. Pedometer-assessed physical activity: measurement and motivations. Presented at the 48th Annual Meeting of the American College of Sports Medicine in Baltimore, MD, May 30–June 3, 2001.

Pate RR, Pratt M, Blair SN, Haskell WL, Macera CA, Bouchard C, et al. Physical activity and public health: a recommendation from the Centers for Disease Control and Prevention and the American College of Sports Medicine. *Journal of the American Medical Association* 273:402–407, 1995.

Krucoff C. 10,000 steps to better health. *Washington Post*, Health section 16, November 23, 1999.

Pronk N. One step at a time: the 10,000 steps program increases physical activity. *Permanente Journal* 7(2):35–36, 2003.

Paffenbarger RS, Wing AL, Hyde RT. Physical activity as an index of heart attack risk in college alumni. *American Journal of Epidemiology* 108:161–175, 1978.

Lee I-M, Sesso HD, Paffenbarger RS. Physical activity and coronary heart disease risk in men: does the duration of exercise episodes predict risk? *Circulation* 102:981–986, 2000.

Bassett DR, Cureton AL, Ainsworth BE. Measurement of daily walking distance: questionnaire versus pedometer. *Medicine and Science in Sports and Exercise* 32:1018–1023, 2000.

Bassett DR, Schneider PL, Huntington GE. Physical activity in an Old Order Amish community. *Medicine and Science in Sports and Exercise* 36:79–85, 2004.

Schneider PL. Accuracy of pedometers and their use in a 10,000 steps per day intervention study (doctoral dissertation). Department of Exercise, Sport, and Leisure Studies, University of Tennessee, Knoxville, 2004.

Feury M. Walk off the weight. *Woman's Day*, 74–78, September 2000.

Thompson DL, Rakow J, Perdue SM. Relationship between accumulated walking and body composition in middle-aged women. *Medicine and Science in Sports and Exercise* 36:911–914, 2004.

Whitt M, Kumanyika S, Bellamy S. Amount and bouts of physical activity in a sample of African-American women. *Medicine and Science in Sports and Exercise* 35:1887–1893, 2003.

Week Four

Lindbergh R. Active living: on the road with the 10,000 Steps program. *Journal of the American Dietetics Association* 100:878–879, 2000.

U.S. Department of Health and Human Services. *Physical Activity and Health: A Report of the Surgeon General*. Atlanta: U.S. Department of Health and Human Services, Centers for Disease Control and Prevention, National Center for Chronic Disease Prevention and Health Promotion, 1996.

Crespo CJ, Keteyian SJ, Heath GW, Sempos CT. Leisure-time physical activity among U.S. adults. *Archives of Internal Medicine* 156:93–98, 1996.

Ainsworth BE, Haskell WL, Whitt MC, Irwin ML, Swartz AM, Strath, S J, et al. Compendium of physical activities: an update of activity codes and MET intensities. *Medicine and Science in Sports and Exercise* 32:S498–S516, 2000.

Oliver J. Pedometer-estimated step rates and energy expenditure. Senior honors project, University of Tennesssee, Knoxville. Spring semester 2004.

Fletcher, C., and Rawlins, C. *The Complete Walker IV.* New York: Knopf Publishing, 2002.

Cary, A. *Parents' Guide to Hiking and Camping: A Trailside Guide.* New York: W. W. Norton and Co., 1997.

Week Five

Howley ET. Energy costs of physical activity. In *Health Fitness Instructor's Handbook,* 4th edition, ET Howley and BD Franks, editors. Champaign, IL: Human Kinetics, 2003.

American College of Sports Medicine. *ACSM's Guidelines for Exercise Testing and Prescription,* 7th edition, M. H. Whaley, senior editor. Philadelphia: Lippincott, Williams, and Wilkins, 2006.

Dwight D. Eisenhower Library. Flexing the nation's muscle: an article about Harry S. Truman. http://eisenhower.archives.gov/truman .html. Last accessed on July 16, 2004.

Harry S. Truman National Historic Site, U.S. Department of Interior National Park Service Collections. www.cr.nps.gov/museum/exhibits/hstr/img.html. Last accessed on July 16, 2004.

Craib M, et al. Physiological test and performance parameters for elite and sub-elite racewalkers. Presented at the American College of Sports Medicine Southeast Regional Meeting, spring 1994.

Fenton RM. Racewalking ground reaction forces. *Sports Biomechanics,* Proceedings of the International Symposium on Biomechanics in Sport, J Terauds, editor, January 1984.

Graves JE, Pollock ML, Montain SJ, Jackson AS, O'Keefe JM. The effect of handheld weights on the physiological responses to walking exercise. *Medicine and Science in Sports and Exercise* 19:260–265, 1987.

Jacobsen BH, Wright T, Dugan B. Load carriage energy expenditure with and without hiking poles during inclined walking. *International Journal of Sports Medicine* 21:356–359, 2000.

Porcari JP, Hendrickson TL, Walter PR, Terry L, Walsko G. The physiological responses to walking with and without Power Poles™ on treadmill exercise. *Research Quarterly for Exercise and Sport* 68:161–166, 1997.

Rodgers CD, VanHeest JL, Schachter CL. Energy expenditure during submaximal walking with Exerstriders®. *Medicine and Science in Sports and Exercise* 27:607–611, 1995.

Jacobson BH, Wright T. A field test comparison of hiking stick use on heartrate and rating of perceived exertion. *Perceptual and Motor Skills* 87:435–438, 1998.

Week Six

Dishman, R. K. *Exercise Adherence: Its Impact on Public Health.* Champaign, IL: Human Kinetics, 1988.

Guiliano, M. *French Women Don't Get Fat.* New York: Alfred A. Knopf, 2004.

Robinson, J. P., and Godbey, G. *Time for Life: The Surprising Ways Americans Use Their Time.* University Park: Pennsylvania State University Press, 1997.

Pucher J, Dijkstra L. Promoting safe walking and cycling to improve public health: lessons from the Netherlands and Germany. *American Journal of Public Health* 93:1509–1516, 2003.

Pucher J, Renne JL. Socioeconomics of urban travel: evidence from the 2001 NHTS. *Transportation Quarterly* 57:49–77, 2003.

Bassett DR, Thompson, DL, Crouter SE, Pucher J. Active transportation and obesity rates in Europe and North America. Submitted for publication, 2005.

International Obesity Task Force (IOTF). European Association for the Study of Obesity. Obesity in Europe: the case for action. www.iotf/media/euobesity.pdf. Last accessed September 2004.

Ewing R, Schmid T, Killingsworth R, Zlot A, Raudenbush S. Relationship between urban sprawl and physical activity, obesity, and morbidity. *American Journal of Health Promotion* 18:47–57, 2003.

Saelens B, Sallis J, Black J, Chen D. Neighborhood-based differences in physical activity: an environment scale evaluation. *American Journal of Public Health* 93:1552–1558, 2003.

Handy SL, Boarnet MG, Ewing R, Killingsworth RE. How the built environment affects physical activity: views from urban planning. *American Journal of Preventive Medicine* 23:64–73, 2002.

Hoehner CM, Brennan LK, Brownson C, Handy SL, Killingsworth R. Opportunities for integrating public health and urban planning approaches to promote active community environments. *American Journal of Health Promotion* 18:14–20, 2003.

Saelens BE, Sallis JF, Frank LD. Environmental correlates of walking and cycling: findings from the transportation, urban design, and planning literatures. *Annals of Behavioral Medicine* 25:80–91, 2003.

How the Authors Hit Their 10,000 Steps a Day

Mark Fenton, 44, engineer, walking expert, father of two. Days range from 7,000 (too much computer) to 15,000 (great hike with the kids), but average 11,000. Walks or bikes his kids to and from school whenever he's not traveling; racewalks (former member and coach of the U.S. team) or runs three days a week for fitness; bikes for most errands around town; kayaks a lot (he counts the step equivalent) for fun; and hikes with the family on conservation land often.

Bonus steps: When speaking at conferences, Mark urges organizers to schedule him to lead morning fitness walks. Then even a full day of meetings doesn't end up stepless!

David Bassett Jr., 47, researcher, professor, father of two. Averages 9,500 steps per day. Jogs around the track at work during lunch breaks (5,000 steps or 3.5 to 4 miles); walks the dog around the neighborhood; hikes with the family in Great Smoky Mountains National Park on weekends; goes for Sunday bike rides.

Bonus steps: Often parks the car, and walks or cycles the rest of the way to work.

Tracy Teare, 39, freelance writer, mother of three. Averages 12,000 steps per day. Cycles, runs, or swims five times a week. Walks the dog, walks with kids to neighborhood waterfall, and plays with them in the yard (current favorite game: red light, green light). Launched a Wednesday Walkers club at her daughters' elementary school.

Bonus steps: Constantly up and down stairs to computer in attic, washer and dryer in basement.

Index

Walking for Health

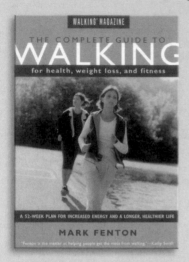

The Complete Guide to Walking

for Health, Fitness, and Weight Loss

By Mark Fenton

ISBN 1-58574-190-6 · $24.95 paperback

Much more than a "how-to" exercise book, *The Complete Guide to Walking* is an interactive handbook that can make the difference for millions of Americans who struggle with weight loss, health and dietary concerns, stress, and chronic fatigue. A former editor at *Walking* magazine, Fenton promises to transform readers of all ages from couch potato to athlete in less than one year with this responsible, motivational, and enjoyable prescription to a healthier life.

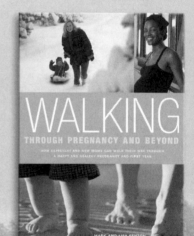

Walking Through Pregnancy and Beyond

How Expectant and New Moms Can Walk Their Way Through a Happy and Healthy Pregnancy and First Year

By Mark Fenton and Lisa Fenton, with Tracy Teare

ISBN 1-59228-384-5 · $19.95 paperback

No more holding back! Research from the experts establishes how much you can and should be exercising while pregnant. Here are personalized walking plans, critical stretching routines, and muscle-strengthening exercises. Anecdotes from real moms, detailed product information on everything from maternity workout clothes to baby carriers, and lots of tips for keeping mom (and later, baby) safe and sound during workouts round out this invaluable guide.

with

The Lyons Press

Available wherever books are sold.
Orders can also be placed on the Web at
www.LyonsPress.com, by phone from
8 A.M. to 5 P.M. at 1-800-243-0495,
or by fax at 1-800-820-2329.

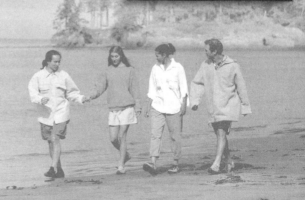